REFLEXOLOGY

Quick Guide to Easy Reflexology Techniques

(The Complete Guide to Reflexology Relieve
Pain and Reduce Tension)

Rosalind Boyd

GW00645393

95000000073226

Published By Rosalind Boyd

Rosalind Boyd

Reflexology: Quick Guide to Easy Reflexology Techniques (The Complete Guide to Reflexology Relieve Pain and Reduce Tension)

ISBN 978-1-77485-425-9

Legal & Disclaimer

The information contained in this book is not designed to replace or take the place of any form of medicine or professional medical advice. The information in this book has been provided for educational and entertainment purposes only.

The information contained in this book has been compiled from sources deemed reliable, and it is accurate to the best of the Author's knowledge; however, the Author cannot guarantee its accuracy and validity and cannot be held liable for any errors or omissions. Changes are periodically made to this book. You must consult your doctor or get professional medical advice before using any of the suggested remedies, techniques, or information in this book.

Upon using the information contained in this book, you agree to hold harmless the Author from and against any damages, costs, and expenses, including any legal fees potentially resulting from the application of any of the information provided by this guide. This disclaimer applies to any damages or injury caused by the use and application, whether directly or indirectly, of any advice or information presented, whether for breach of contract, tort, negligence, personal injury, criminal intent, or under any other cause of action.

You agree to accept all risks of using the information presented inside this book. You need to consult a professional medical practitioner in order to ensure you are both able and healthy enough to participate in this program.

TABLE OF CONTENTS

Introduction

The practice of the reflexology field has been practiced for a long time and has been proven to assist sufferers of stress and pain live more fulfilling lives. It is not a replacement for traditional medicine, but rather is an addition to traditional treatments to help patients manage.

When you practice reflexology and apply it correctly , you can benefit from many issues it can assist with such as backaches teethaches, headaches and sore throats stomach pains, knee pains kidney issues, and the list goes on. When you look at the foot and hand charts for the first time , showing the pathways of the nerves that connect to other parts of your body, you'll be astonished.

Find out how far back in time this concept was used in the past and then how this was introduced to the present through medical pioneers. Discover how it affects different systems in the body and the basic principles that enable it to work.

As you go through the book, you will begin to learn about the best techniques to treat common ailments, broaden your mind and focus on your body in the way you are aware of how it requires attention. There is nobody who understands the body in the same way as you. It doesn't matter if you have discomfort to make use of reflexology. There are reflexes that generally help you to have a better health for your physique and an improved mind.

When you have mastered the basics and techniques in this book, you'll be inspired to share the information with your family and friends. So , without further ado, enjoy reading and be healthy!

Chapter 1: Fundamentals of Reflexology

The History of Reflexology

Reflexology wasn't introduced to the West until the late 20th century, even though it is known the practice was prevalent by the early Chinese, Egyptian, and Indian culture. The oldest records date back to 2,500 B.C. inside the grave of Egyptian Physician Ankhmahor. Inside the tomb , a picture was found that depicts two men working with their feet and hands of two other men on the pictograph. The pictograph is surrounded by hieroglyphics. it was decoded to be "do not allow it to be painful" and the reply "I do what you like".

It is believed that the Northern American Indians are believed to have been practicing a kind of reflexology for many centuries. Hand and foot therapy in China could date to as early as 4000 B.C. If the great minds of the medical profession in the West had not asked about this type of treatment, it may not have been presented to the world.

The first individuals from the West to promote this method of treatment to the West was Dr. William Fitzgerald; an expert in ear, nose and throat specialist in ear, nose and throat. He is credited as the creator of the reflexology technique called "Zone Therapy". In his own study, he discovered the fact that when pressure is applied to specific regions of the body, it could cause an anesthetic reaction in other areas of the body.

He further elaborated on his discovery and separated parts of the body into 10 zones which begin at to the top of your head to the soles of the feet. He found that when he applied pressure with a band that was placed on the middle of finger of the patient or by putting clamps on the fingers' tips of the patient, the patient was able to undergo minor operations without the use of an anesthesia. This was an extremely controversial procedure for the time.

Another person who could play an important role in introduction of reflexology in people in the West included

Eunice Ingham. Within the United States she has often been called "The The Mother of Modern Reflexology". She worked in a doctor's clinic as a physiotherapist, and developed her ideas on her work with Dr. Fitzgerald's Zone Therapy. She was of the opinion that the therapy might be more effective when done with feet instead of hands.

With this in mind, she created a map of the whole foot, stating that the foot is an image to the human body. She took a unique method of presenting her findings and travelled across America for 30 years, teaching her techniques to nurses, doctors and other practitioners of reflexology. She wrote two books, and also developed charts and theories known as The Ingham Method that are the basis for reflexology throughout the West until today. It is believed that the International Institute of Reflexology still continues to carry on the work she did. She continued to work and be an innovator until the age of 80 at which point she took a break. She died in 1974 aged eighty-five.

Reflexology: The Simple Basics of Reflexology

The practice of reflexology involves applying pressure to certain areas on the feet, hands and ears. Reflexology generally is an exercise in relaxation so that stress is relieved and relief may be discovered for specific types of pain.

It is believed that regions where the stress is applied is linked directly to certain organs and functions in the body. The people who use this method and trust in the benefits, feel the pressure is responsible for actions within the organs and systems involved and thus generating beneficial effects for the body.

A reflexologist who is practicing will adhere to a chart of the foot or hand or ear while applying pressure to certain locations to relieve some of the ailments that patients experience. They do not just employ their hands for applying pressure but can also employ bamboo sticks, rubber balls made of wood and rubber bands. People who practice reflexology may find themselves in areas that deal with physical therapy and massage and chiropractics. This is believed as a safe method of treatment. However be aware that with the use of a vigorous pressure can cause discomfort.

the benefits of Practicing Reflexology

There are many benefits, both mental and health wise , that come as a result of reflexology. In this section , you'll be able to learn about the potential benefits that you can reap from reflexology.

Increased Function of the Nerves As we age, along with aging , there are certain changes to our bodies. One of the changes is that nerves start to be less sensitive, especially around the extremities. Reflexology has been proven to connect more than 7,000 different nerves in a single session. This has improved their response and function. Nerves are thought to be a neural pathway. However like muscles, they require work on occasion to keep functioning.

More Energy Levels - by re-aligning the roles between muscles and organs within

the body; metabolism can be increased and energy levels increased by reflexology.
Better Circulation: It has been established that reflexology can boost circulation in the body, which means that blood and oxygen be able to flow more easily through the body and, consequently, the proper amounts of blood and oxygen are reaching essential organs. It also leads to quicker healing, and damaged cells can grow with greater speed.

Relaxation - As mentioned in the past, reflexology may unblock to clear the pathways of neural activity, which can create a sense of peace throughout your body and lower stress levels. It is often employed to treat insomnia and other sleep disorders due to the fact that it helps your body recover the state of relaxation and help people get back into their regular sleeping routine.

Eliminates Toxins that reflexology aids in the process of elimination of toxins is to aid in the function of gall bladder as well as aid in eliminating urinary tract infections. This helps the body better rid itself of toxins and waste.

stimulates the Nervous System Through opening up the neural pathways, the central nervous system is stimulated. This has amazing effects on a variety of aspects. For instance, through this type of stimulation , the brain becomes awake and can process input with greater efficiency. This means it will enhance cognitive capacity, improve memory, and ultimately perform better.

Treatment of headaches and migraines If you feel tension on specific muscles, it could be the reason for migraines and headaches. By applying pressure at the appropriate places reflexology can alleviate or eliminate discomfort that is associated with migraines and headaches. Stress-related headaches are also eliminated since it relieves the psychological stress that is the cause of discomfort. This is among the primary reasons why people do reflexology.

Speedier Healing Time - Because of the increase in activity in the nerves and improved circulation, cells are able to grow faster , which reduces on the time it takes to heal injuries. If there is physical limitation because of injury, the higher energy levels may make people more excited to start treatment to get back on their feet.

Cancer Relief Reflexology is not making any claim for cancer treatment or cure for cancer; however, it can assist with the negative side consequences of the disease. When patients undergo chemotherapy, they typically experience symptoms of nausea and vomiting. They also have difficulty sleeping, or digestive issues and reflexology can ease these symptoms. There is research underway which could suggest that due to the improvement in circulation and the elimination of neural pathways, the growth of cancerous cells may be slowed down and increase the antioxidant activity that are associated with chemotherapy.

Pregnancy - Due to its ability to ease stress and boost circulation reflexology can aid women in avoiding post-partum depression as well as have quicker recovery time after having a baby. This can also have an impact on the necessity for pain medication during labor as well as the duration of the actual labor.

There are many who don't believe or aren't convinced that reflexology is effective and have the right to express their opinions. The fact that it's been in use for many thousands of years and is aiding many people is proof that their beliefs are not valid. Reflexology isn't claiming as a cure to all the ailments of the world, butit can be used as a complement to aid in other therapies that are needed.

Chapter 2: Reflexology for Hands and Feet

General Hand Reflexology

Hand reflexology is for majority used to relieve headaches, constipation and discomforts in the shoulder region. In this part of the book, you'll learn about the general use and procedure of hand reflexology. Later, the details of the techniques that are used to use for specific purposes will be covered in greater detail.

If you are beginning to do the hand reflexology you do,, you must remember that when you work with the hands, more intense pressure is needed. The reason why you should apply more forceful pressure on your hands is due to the fact that the reflex points you wish to access are more deep in the hands than the feet.

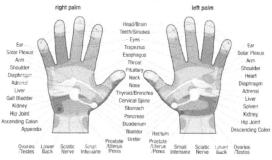

Hand Reflexology Chart

Find a comfortable seat to relax in, preferred in a space with minimal light to create a relaxing ambience.

Relax yourself by applying a tiny amount of your preferred cream on the palms of your hands. Lavender is a wonderful choice since it is renowned for its relaxing properties. The use of lotion isn't common in an expert reflexology session however, in a try it yourself session , it could aid in relaxing. It's also possible to choose oil if that's your preference over lotions, however, ensure it's an oil that absorbs into the skin, and not make your hands slick. It is also important to select one that is absorbed completely.

* To unwind yourself and your hands, rub the lotion until it's completely absorption.

13

A few minutes of gentle massage can help let your hands relax and will allow them to be more flexible for the massage you'll be performing.

* Close your eyes and concentrate on the area of your body where you are experiencing pain or perhaps it is just an area of your body that isn't in alignment Focus on the specific region.

* Check the chart for your reflexology to determine the hand point where you should apply pressure to the body part. The reading of these charts will be discussed in the next part of the book.

* You must press hard on the spot identified by the chart to activate the reflex your body requires. Press hard, but when you start feeling discomfort, you can reduce the pressure a bit.

* Keep the pressure in place for a period of 30 seconds, then release.

* Wait some time before applying pressure again to the point. Following the pressure application, you may continue the pressure application for thirty seconds

or choose to press and release quickly, in a rapid pulsing motion for 30 minutes.

* If applying pressure the normal method is too painful for you, try pressing the pressure point in a gentler method using the following method. Utilize your forefinger or thumb to gently massaging the pressure point in an upward move for five second. afterwards reverse that circular motion after five seconds. Repeat the circular massage for multiple sections, making sure to turn the motion around after every 5 seconds.

* During your exercise, you should attempt to hit all pressure points on your hands at least once. However you should keep your attention on the areas you're having difficulty with at the moment.

After you have finished your session, you must take a break and sit for at least 10 minutes. If possible, to reap the best benefits from the reflexology, take your time to rest for around a half an hour.

* In the next few hours following your session consume a few glass of water. This will help eliminate the toxins released by

your organs and muscles in your reflexology session.

The Hand Reflexology Technique and Safety

Here are some suggestions to remember when performing hand reflexology for yourself or even on a person you know.

A. You can get the same results with hand reflexology just as you would by applying it to any other body part but the results typically take a more time.

B. In the theory of hand reflexology, it is said that if there is a problem within the body, the pressure point on the hand will be different. The point may feel tender, soft and more difficult than normal as well as painful fingertips. If you notice this occurring, refer to your hand reflexology chart identify which part within your body that it could be.

C. If you're doing your exercise, make sure you utilize both hands to be sure you're maintaining the balance of your body and not causing any other thing to get out of balance.

Do. It is suggested to practice your sessions in dimly lit rooms however, you are able to perform reflexology at your desk or traveling on an airplane.

A. If you are planning to conduct sessions for a person you know Sit them in front of each other at the tables and have their hands placed on a towel. This will allow them to keep their hands relaxed.

F. If you're an arthritis sufferer and you find it too difficult to apply pressure, consider using different items. It is not necessary to spend money on expensive reflexology tools and there are many items at your house that you can use. Golf balls are an excellent example. Try by squeezing it into your hands. If it is difficult for you, place your ball down on tabletop or flat surface. Then place your hands on top. press as hard as you can comfortably and move the ball to hit the pressure points of your hands.

Warnings about Hand Reflexology

Although reflexology is a secure addition to various kinds of treatments, there are some things to take into consideration.

A. If you suffer from an injury to your hand, you should stay clear of the hand reflexology, and instead make use of other parts of your body for reflexology like your feet or your ears.

B. Reflexology is meant as a supplement to conventional treatments and therapies. Don't try using reflexology to diagnose an illness or condition, and do not apply it as the sole method of treatment.

General Foot Reflexology

Reflexology on the feet is an approach to alleviate the many ailments the body may be suffering However before you start doing private sessions for yourself, it is important to understand the procedure. In this section , the fundamental techniques of foot reflexology are covered so that you can have more understanding before you start your sessions.

A. Before beginning the treatment, and to make your feet more comfortable, spend some time in an enjoyable foot soak. It will relax the feet and make them more open for the therapy.

B. After drying your feet, locate a comfy spot to sit on the ground; you can Try using an exercise mat in order to help you feel more comfortable. It is best to do this inside a dimly-lit space. You could also add some aromatherapy candles that will make your ambience to be more peaceful.

C. The room's temperature should be comfortable, not too hot but also not cold. The focus should be on the practice of reflexology and not on the temperature of the room.

D. With a peppermint foot cream, gentle massage your feet in order to let them relax until the lotion is fully in the body. Relaxing your feet prior to starting, you'll be able to get the best results from your reflexology treatment.

E. Choose which foot you want to start with and then cover the other foot with a thin cover to ensure it is warm and comfortable.

F. Shut your eyes and unwind your thoughts let it go, relax and concentrate on the region of your body you'd like to focus on during your exercise.

G. Check your foot reflexology chart in order to find out what the location of your pressure point is you must focus on.

H. Press into the pressure point for thirty seconds , then release. Give a couple of seconds before pressing the pressure point again. Continue to repeat the 30 second hold, or pulsate it by pressing and then releasing in five second intervals over an entire thirty seconds.

I. Work through your whole foot before moving to the next foot.

J. After the session has ended, you should take ten minutes to sit down and relax. If time permits , you can take an hour of rest following the session.

K. The next couple of hours , drink lots of water to rid you of the waste discharged during your session.

Foot Reflexology Tips and Warns

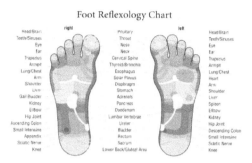

Foot Reflexology Chart

A. Certain people have difficulty to perform foot reflexology on themselves due to their inability to grasp their foot toes. It is essential to locate a position that's comfortable enough to do the pressure application or else it'll be useless. If you are unable to locate a position that feels comfortable , ask your partner or someone else to assist you. You should be sure to return the favor , so that they be healthier too.

B. If you're struggling to relax, listen to some gentle relaxing music with a low volume.

Warns

A. Don't strain to get to your feet. This can cause other issues. If you are unable to perform the task and do not have a partner, take a look at going to an experienced reflexologist.

B. Like hand reflexology, this is a form of supplementary of treatment. Do not attempt to diagnose a medical problem to treat the problem by foot reflexology. It is a method that is meant to be used in conjunction with the traditional treatment options to treat your ailments.

Chapter 3: What is the reason and How Reflexology is Beneficial for the body

The hand or foot has imaginary lines that separate them into sections that reflect on the human body. The body is split into systems based on physiology. this can be seen in the feet and hands. The reflexes that are found in feet and hands directly link to the systems of the body. Each of these systems is part of a larger organic system that allows the body to work the way it does.

The effects on The Skeletal and the Muscular System

Whatever the system within the body, it is subject to stimulation. Based on the stimulus source, the results can be positively or negatively. Through reflexology, the body is taught to respond with positive energy, which can allow us to react in innovative and essential ways to stress. To manage stress, one needs to let go. Once stress is gone, it becomes apparent how life is viewed and effectively through natural processes to reach objectives.

The muscles in your body hold stress and reflexology work on the musculature of your body to help it let go of tension and ease the tension. By regularly practicing reflexology, your muscular system as well as your bones will demonstrate that it's working with less pains and aches throughout your body. Reflexology operates from the inside of the body, stimulating the systems to start healing instead of working on only one region as in traditional treatments. When muscles start to loosen,, the nervous system kicks in and assist by dissolving blockages and constrictions.

The effects on the Circulatory and Nervous Systems.

If you perform reflexology, the nervous system gets affected in a direct and indirect way. The hands and feet are equipped with nerve pathways that are stimulated by reflexes which communicate with the bigger system to establish the direction that leads to and from the central nervous system.

The feet and hands during reflexology, it directly affects blood vessels, which stimulates the circulation system. In addition, it indirectly stimulates other nerves, too. At this point, other sensory systems like your skin , also your sense organs such as the ears, mouth, nose and eyes are affected. When reflexes in your feet or hands are stimulated during a session , the skin transmits signals to other body systems. When considering the concept of reflexology, the hands and feet can be thought of as sensory organs.

Each body system is affected by reflexology. When systems are affected by contact, the reflexology can stimulate the nervous system by triggering the sensation. Nervous system in contact with all parts of the body, so reflexology is believed as the pathway to all other systems that are able to align the body to the how it ought to be.

Reflexology's functions within the body

By utilizing the different organs within the body, reflexology is able to stimulate vital energy forces within the body. These vital energies help the body perform just as it was created to. The fundamental duties of reflexology are as the following.

* Controlling the regular bodily functions of the body.
* Enhancing one's overall health.
* Increases circulation via stimulation.
* It helps to bring one into a state calm.
* Relieves pain from emotional and physical traumas.
* Aids in reducing the amount of medicines the body is dependent on.
* Helps with internal communication between different systems in the body.

When the reflexology functions are carried out, it triggers reactions. When the bodily responses are stimulated by reflexology, the positive effects will begin to be felt. When you improve your body, your mind will also improve. As your mind begins to improve, you'll begin to think more positive and as you become more positive in your thinking, you'll experience better emotional well-being. When your mood improves, you'll notice that you are more cheerful and feel more joyful, and a greater appreciation of life will help you to be more confident. As you attain this greater happiness in your life, it comes spiritual happiness and that is accompanied by improved health in general.

Chapter 4: Five Specific DIY Foot Reflexology Techniques

1. Foot reflexology is a treatment for headaches and Migraines - Headaches as well as migraines can result from many factors like stress, working too hard and major changes to your life, or allergies. It isn't important what the reason is, the most important thing is to eliminate the discomfort that can be difficult to bear. Check out the below chart. The reflex points where you'll be working are highlighted for you.

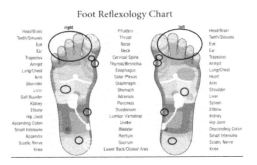

Foot Reflexology Chart

Moving through the spine to treat Headaches and Migraines

Treatment of the spine is the best way to begin treatment for migraines and headaches. The primary treatment should focus on the upper part of the spine, around the neck. This will allow tension to be eased and reduce the discomfort. Reflexology can provide relief even if you're not sure about the root of the migraine or headache. Follow these steps for the initial method of using reflexology to ease headaches and migraine pain.

A. When you are sitting, utilize the left side of your hand help support your left foot.

B. With your left hand start with your biggest toe, and then gently massage the top of your three toes. If you're experiencing an acute migraine , your toes could be a little sensitive; then press them lightly. Apply pressure and massage your three toes for 5 minutes.

C. Switch feet and make use of your thumb on the right side to perform the procedure with your left hand.

D. On both feet, utilize your thumbs or your knuckles and press the reflex points on the bottom of your toes, both on the top of your foot and the sole. look up the foot chart to find points of reflex.

Your toes are the place where all reflex points are that influence the sinuses the head, brain and neck that could be the main cause of your migraine or headache issue.

Moving through the liver for Migraines and Headaches

In many instances, migraines and headaches can be traced to digestive system, therefore optimizing the functioning the liver plays is crucial. Your liver plays a significant impact on your health and general well-being. In reality, the majority of humanity lives a life of exposing their livers to fats pesticides, drugs chemicals, food additives and beverages, but however, not all of it is done so. By using reflexology, you can begin healing your liver while you ease the pain of migraine or headache.

A. When you are sitting, make use of your hands to hold the upper part on your left foot. Since your liver is situated on the right side of your body, you'll only be working your right foot. Utilize the left hand to press on the liver reflex, that runs straight down from your big toe and under the ball of your foot. Refer to this chart to get more information on the reflex point.

B. Utilizing your thumb, you can move all the pressure points, starting from the inside of your foot and moving along the direction of the ball until it reaches the outside.

C. Work towards returning to your initial starting point by applying pressure as you go back.

The Cervical Spine to treat Headaches and Migraines

Inside your feet has curves that resemble the spine. Through this method of reflexology, you'll focus on the cervical region of the spine in order to treat the pain that comes from migraine or headache.

A. Sitting in a comfortable position in a sitting position, place your right foot with your left. With your left thumb, apply pressure on the point where your foot's big toe joins the rest of your foot. Apply pressure to the reflex point for a period of time.

B. Consult your foot reflex chart , and go through the various points that are connected to your spine.

C. Repeat the process with the reverse direction on your left side.

2. Foot Reflexology to Lose Weight The loss of weight appears to be among the most important concerns for most people in the present day. When you practice reflexology, your body can be stimulated in many ways to aid in the fight against weight loss. Reflexology can be a wonderful method to add to your diet regimen and is also a secure method to help you reach your goals. If you are using reflexology for weight loss, you'll be working with the points for the stomach, spleen and the pancreas, gallbladder and the glands of the endocrine system, as well as the relaxing points. When each point is explained, you will be able to understand how it can aid in losing weight. See the following chart for better location of pressure points.

Utilizing the Spleen to help with Weight Loss

In stimulating the spleen by reflexology, your appetite will be decreased, which will make you want to eat less food, which helps in losing weight.

A. Sitting in a seated position, utilize the right side of your hand in order to hold the left side of your foot. The left thumb to massage the spleen reflex point , which is located at the bottom of your foot, beneath the ball of the foot in a straight line from the space between the small toe and the fourth approximately one half inch out from outside the feet. Check out the chart to get more information.

B. It is recommended to apply pressure for minimum five minutes per day.

C. Repeat the process with the other foot.

Work through The Stomach and Pancreas to Lose Weight

When you are dieting, you will likely eat less food. Through working the reflexes of the stomach and pancreas , you stimulate your body, ensuring that it absorbs greater nutrients in the foods you eat and ensure that you get the most benefit from your food you consume.

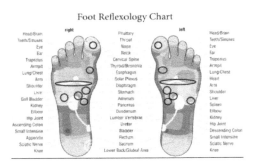

Foot Reflexology Chart

A. Begin by sitting and place your left foot with the palm of your left hand. Make use of your thumb in order to press down on every of the points. As you apply pressure , move towards the outside of your foot, and when you have reached the limit, apply pressure to the other direction.

B. Repeat the process with the other foot.

Utilizing the Gallbladder to lose weight

The gallbladder stores Bile, which is released by the liver in order to break down fats that are accumulated from food that is not digested. This aids in losing weight challenge.

A. In a sitting position, cradle your right foot into your left hand since this is the point where the reflex for the gallbladder is located. Apply your thumb's pressure to the reflex point , and keep it for a few minutes.

B. Repeat the process on the other foot.

Utilizing The Endocrine Glands for Weight Loss

Stress can play a key factor for the successful or failure of a diet plan and by working on the pituitary gland thyroid gland along with the adrenal gland through reflexology, you can deal with stress more effectively and stand an increased chance of success.

A. With the help of the chart, go through the reflex points on the feet to reap the benefits of reflexology.

B. Utilize the opposite hand to support your foot as you do your best to ensure that you are comfortable and at ease.

Moving through relaxation for weight Loss

Sleeping well is a crucial factor in the successful weight loss process and through the use of reflexology techniques to relax, you'll be able to enjoy a better nights sleep.

A. Begin by using your left foot. utilize your right thumb to place it across the diaphragm lines starting from inside and ending on the exterior of your foot. Put your left thumb on the lower joints between your feet. As you press with your middle finger, you can gently move your toes forward and back across one's left thumb.

3. Foot Reflexology to help with constipation It's a topic which people do not like to discuss, but it's an integral part of daily life. Reflexology isn't cure for constipation in the long term but it could aid in occasional discomfort that it causes. If you're suffering with chronic constipation, you must consult with your doctor. If you follow the steps below, you should be able manage constipation-related bouts.

A. If you're constipated, there's a high possibility that you don't have enough fluids to move the waste through therefore, make sure you make sure you drink plenty of water prior to starting your workout.

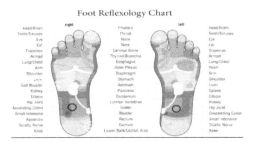

Foot Reflexology Chart

B. Begin with the foot you prefer and make use of your thumb opposite to trigger those reflex points.

C. Make a thumb-walk through the space between the large and small intestines with both feet. It's similar to the pulse but you'll keep the pressure for a little longer before you move on.

D. Change between feet to foot until you've completed the procedure at minimum five times per foot. It should take between 10 and 15 minutes.

4. Foot Reflexology to help with a Cold There's nothing more frustrating than having a million tasks to complete and then being slow-going due to a nagging cold. A cold isn't necessarily the most serious issue to be concerned about, but they can place a huge impact on your productivity according to the severity. Reflexology isn't the only remedy for the common cold however, it can help bring you back to work. If your symptoms are getting worse, it is recommended to see your physician and continue using reflexology as an adjunct to treatment.

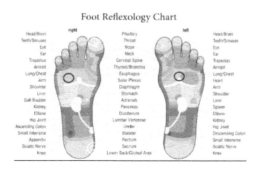

Foot Reflexology Chart

The Lungs, the Workout and the Chest to treat a cold

They are also the primary defense against harmful pathogens that could infect the body. Working with the reflex points of the lungs can aid in the healing process from an illness. If you are using reflexology to treat colds, try these guidelines to get a better outcome.

It is best to do it the moment you wake up.

* Make sure to do it an hour prior to or following your lunch.

* Make sure to do it at the time at the end of your working day.

* Make it a priority to do this before you go to bed.

These are the moments that will provide you the results you're seeking.

A. Your thumb will be used in order to massage and apply pressure over the whole surface in the lung reflex. This should be done for at minimum five minutes at least two times each day.

B. Repeat the process with the other foot.

C. When you notice an area that's more tender, try pushing the area further and massaging it more intensely. Within the reason.

When you examine the chart, you could notice that there are additional regions that are afflicted by the cold. you could include these points in your appointment as well. This can include the nasal passages, sinuses, throat eye, neck and any other part which is experiencing discomfort as a result of cold.

5. Foot Reflexology for relieving Sciatica Pain - Sciatica pain in your lower back can drag your down and stop you from completing your tasks. Through foot reflexology, you'll be able to alleviate the discomfort and return to your feet. When it comes to back pain, this treatment is not just focused on Sciatic nerve, but also on Sciatic nerve. It will also consider other back that may result from or cause Sciatica pain.

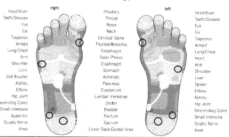

Foot Reflexology Chart

A. To get started working on the sciatic pain, start by working on your cervical spine.

B. When you are sitting, make use of the left hand of your body to hold the foot of the left. With your thumb from the right hand, begin at the point that the big toe connects with the foot. Press to the point and then run it along the outside of the foot, aiming to trigger all the reflex points that are located on the back. It is important to note that the points you're trying to activate are not located on the sole of your foot however, they are along the inner edge.

C. Repeat on the opposite foot and then move to the next.

D. Then spend some time doing exercises with the sciatic nerve. It is recommended to apply pressure starting at the beginning and then move it around until you are just below the ankle bone, which is located on the outside of your foot. This will help increase blood flow and get circulation improving to ease the discomfort. Repeat the process on both feet.

A. When working on the upper back, shoulder points should be applied pressure both on the top and sole of your foot. While working with the sole your foot, make sure you apply pressure to the sole of your foot and do not put too much pressure on the top of your foot. Repeat the procedure across both feet a similar length of time in order to maintain your balance.

Now you know how to use foot reflexology on yourself in order to help with some of the frequent ailments sufferers experience. When you study the chart, you will see that there are many more reflexes which can be utilized to boost happiness and decrease the pain and stress. In the the next chapter, five strategies to treat hand reflexology are discussed to enhance your understanding and improve your overall health.

Chapter 5: Five Hand Reflexology

Methods that are DIY

In this chapter , you're going to master five hand reflexology strategies which you can use at the home, on the plane, and even at your workplace desk. Reflexology was created for the feet and hands by using the nerves of both to relay signals to the body to ensure that it functions to its best. Learn how easy it is to feel more relaxed within a ˋmatter of minutes by using reflexology for the hand.

6. Hand Reflexology to treat menstrual cramps Women across the world are suffering from cramps in their menstrual cycle. Through hand reflexology, women can reduce the pain and discomfort that comes with their cycle. Take a look at the chart below which has been highlighted to highlight the points of reflexology that work to relieve menstrual cramps.

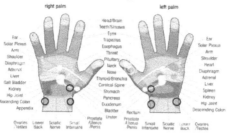

Hand Reflexology Chart

A. Select the hand you would like to begin with, and place it gently on the palm of the other hand.

B. With fingers of your other hand apply pressure on the reflex points and keep it for 30 minutes. After a few seconds, repeat the procedure five times for each point. It is also possible to massage the area using your thumb if it feels too uncomfortable for you.

C. Switch hands, then repeat the process over and over.

D. Continue to practice reflexology at least twice per day until your flow has diminished.

7. Hand Reflexology to Relieve the Hip Pain As we age , we discover some areas that begin to hurt and more. Hand

reflexology can be used to ease hip pain
for just a few minutes each day.

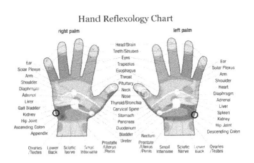

Hand Reflexology Chart

A. Put your left hand into the palm of your
left hand for support.

B. Use your thumb on your left hand for
applying pressure on the reflex point by
using the palm of your hand to support it
and increase the pressure.

C. For thirty seconds, then hold for
another couple of seconds, then repeat.
To get the best results , try at minimum
five times.

D. Switch hands and repeat the procedure.

8. Hand Reflexology for better sleep
There's nothing more frustrating than
having to wake up earlier in the day, and
you can't sleep. Do a hand reflexology

session on the nights you aren't sleeping and end up sleeping well within a matter of minutes. If you are working towards a better sleep, you'll be working on the diaphragm reflex , as shown in the graph below.

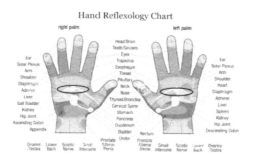

Hand Reflexology Chart

A. Find a comfortable place to relax and lie down.

B. With the left hand, place the right hand into the cradle.

C. Utilizing the thumb of your left hand, massage the the diaphragm line across the body from one point to the next. Repeat this several times before switching hands to repeat the procedure.

You could also try this for your partner's feet when they're having a tough sleeping in the night. They will be grateful for the help.

9. Hand Reflexology to treat high blood pressure It is a medical issue which is becoming more prevalent. Hand reflexology isn't a cure for the problem and is not recommended as a substitute for traditional medical treatment. However it could be utilized as an adjunct treatment to treat the issue. If you are trying to lower blood pressure, there are many reflex points to focus on during a session , which you can see on the chart below.

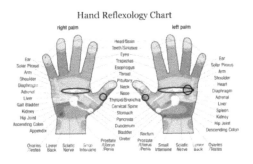

Hand Reflexology Chart

A. Beginning by using the left hand is an excellent choice since this is the hand actually has the heart reflex on.

B. Place your hand on the left with your right and then press it to the heart's reflex. For 30 seconds, hold and then let it go. After a few seconds, apply the pressure again and hold for 30 seconds. Repeat for five times.

C. Utilize your right thumb to apply to press and then move it across the diaphragm line from inside of your hand towards the outside and then return. Repeat this several times.

D. Then, turn your hand towards the palm-down position. Find your reflex spot of your thyroid gland between your thumb and fore fingers of the right hand . press. For 30 seconds, then let it go for a few seconds , and repeat 5 times.

E. Switch hands, and then repeat the procedure in the direction of the thyroid gland, as well as diaphragm.

10. Hand Reflexology is a great treatment for Tooth Aches - A tooth pain can be one of the most painful pains in the world. It

can make the whole body hurt and you'd like it to go away. Hand reflexology isn't an alternative to visiting the dentist, but it can assist in dealing with discomfort until you get there.

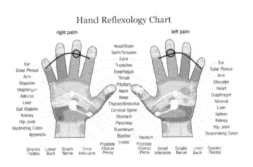

Hand Reflexology Chart

A. The teeth's reflexes extend across the four fingers of each hand.

B. By using fingers and thumbs on the opposite hand , apply pressure to the reflex point on each finger. Hold for 30 seconds. Repeat the process on the fingers five times prior to switching hands.

C. Repeat the entire procedure on the reverse side.

Now you have the necessary knowledge to deal with many of the most prevalent discomforts. The best benefit of hand reflexology or more specifically, the fact that it is effective, is the fact that it can perform it anyplace. If your tooth hurts when you're at work, you can spend a few minutes at your desk to have the treatment and help ease the pain.

Chapter 6: The Fundamentals about

Reflexology

Have you ever believed that your body is able to self-heal? This is one of the many amazing abilities that many are prone to overlook, particularly in these days, when there appears to be a cure or facility that is able to treat nearly all health issues. There are instances where it is best to verify this claim. It is possible to allow the healing process to take place in a natural way or discover ways to make use of alternative forms of healing, such as reflexology.

Reflexology, in addition to being an alternative form of medical treatment, is also referred to as a healing art that is natural. It is based on the notion that your body has reflexes on the feet and hands that correspond to each part of your body. It is essential to locate these reflexes, activate them the muscles, and then apply pressure in order to increase the function and rid yourself of any pain that every of your body parts are experiencing.

If you only take the time to look around your hands and feet, they are more sensitive than you imagine them to be. The body parts of your feet and hands can sense the movement of your body, alignment of weight stretching, pressure and alignment.

Reflexology and its Effects

This type of alternative medicine is best handled by a doctor who has been trained on the pressure points within the body. It is also possible to do it yourself using certain tools that can help you locate the pressure spots. The next step is to be able to use your fingers and thumbs in order to activate these pressure points, and to target the body parts that are connected to them.

What is it that's not?

Although reflexology is used extensively all over the world as a complement to other treatments for different ailments, it's not intended to treat or diagnose any illness. It is typically used to prevent illness for health issues, particularly which include diabetes, anxiety kidney disease, PMS, asthma and migraine.

This form of alternative medicine has received more interest from all over the globe. In Denmark there have been studies that show that using reflexology has resulted in less absenteeism and sick leave from employees. Denmark has employed reflexologists within their municipal and corporate offices from the start of the 1990s. They have increased the amount of productivity for employees, which can translate into financial savings to employers.

Learning how to recognize Reflexology Points as well as Areas

There are specific areas and points which are located in the feet, hands and face that correspond with various organs and body parts. This is the first step you must master through practice - to determine the location of these areas and points are, and to which body part they connect to. Professionals have also used diagrams of the reflex point which are available in a variety of shapes and are made of different materials.

While certain practitioners describe the minor reflex points in different ways however, the majority of practitioners have a common understanding of the most important reflex points within the body. If you visit an expert, you will be asked about the issues that bother you, so that the practitioner can find the points that relate to the issue. He will then work on your entire body, before making a focus on the problem areas.

If you're getting caught up in the rush and are in a state of anxiety, you'll probably receive a relaxing session. In this scenario the reflexologist will be working in your ears for a while until you're nerves have settled down. The primary goal is to relieve the tension or strain on your nervous system , and achieve the proper energy balance.

Reflexology in Relation to Other Therapies

Reflexology is often thought of as being associated with two other kinds of alternative medicine: Acupressure and acupuncture. These therapies all work by stimulating the key points in the body that draw out the energy that is needed and attempt to ease any issue the patient suffers from. There could be some commonalities however some pressure points used in acupuncture or acupressure do not align in the same way as the reflexes in the map of reflexology.

Acupressure practitioners can trace around 800 reflexes which traverse the entire body, and are located on meridians. These are the energy lines that are thin and long. lines that are affixed to the entire body.

Reflexology can also be misunderstood with another type alternative treatment that is called massage. Both employ contact, but in various methods. Massage can relax muscles through specific techniques, like tapping, kneading and friction.

Reflexology is not based on the same techniques used in massage. Instead, it uses what's called micro-movements. Instead of large and powerful motions like those in a massage practitioners walk and then grasp the reflex points with the finger or thumb until your body reacts to the movement. Massage therapists work on the outside of your body in order to deal with your issue in the interior and the reverse is performed by the reflexologist.

This stimulates the nerve system activating the points within your body to influence and affect its outer zones. You'll be fully clothed during a session of reflexology but this is not the case with massage, as the therapist must apply ointments or oils to treat the external regions that are located on your body.

A Short Look at its history

It is difficult to determine since it has been practiced since the time of the first civilizations. The theory is that the practice was handed down down through generations through oral traditions. There were instances in the past when pictographs were used to implement this method are documented. For instance there were impressions of feet found in the Egyptian tomb in Ankhamor during 2330 BC.

A book, which was regarded as an important classic in China called"The Golden Emperor's Classic of Internal Medicine, includes a chapter devoted to the various points found on feet and how they affect the body in general. The book was written around the year 1000 BC.

Within the US, William H. Fitzgerald, MD is often called the founder of this type of alternative medical treatment. It is because of the book he wrote in 1917 that discussed those 10 vertical areas across the body. It also discussed the ways to identify an injury and ease it with pressure applied to correct locations and points.

A lot of doctors and practitioners continue to research and apply this technique throughout the years. One example is the Dr. Shelby Riley expanded the studies of Dr. Fitzgerald. In the end, Dr. Riley was able to develop the precise diagram of reflex points of the feet and hands.

Doctor. Riley worked closely with the physiotherapist Eunice Ingham. She carried on the research and discovered that the most sensitive and responsive to pressure points is the feet. Ingham invented the foot maps, which remain in use until the present. She also created the reflexology chart, which is effective and well-known to this day. The chart was refined by her niece, Dwight Byers, who is employed in the International Reflexology Institute.

The map of reflex points within the ear was first recorded by Dr. Paul Nogier in 1957. Since then, the map has been subject to growth and improvements and is being used by a variety of practitioners and those who are interested.

Chapter 7: Therapeutic Effects of

Reflexology

What effects does reflexology have on the body? How can you profit from the stimulation of the reflex zones?

1. Benefits of neurophysiology

The nervous system gets greatest from pressure applied to your hands and feet as you experience the therapeutic touch of reflexology. Studies are currently being conducted to demonstrate the connection between the nervous system and the endocrine as well as immune system.

At present, the most evident benefits of reflexology which fall within this category are normalization of heart rates, as well as feeling more relaxed and content. It also increases the energy levels of your body and helps you to get a good night's sleep. This can make you feel more confident about yourself generally. It also helps increase your respiration and digestion and lower the level of anxiety and stress.

2. Increased lymphatic and vascular circulation

There was a study in Japan which was conducted in the late 90s, and showed that this type alternative medicine could improve the circulation of blood in the legs. This is particularly beneficial to those who are stiff or who have trouble walking or getting around. Therapeutic foot massages have the capability of lowering both diastolic as well as systolic blood pressure. It also assists in reducing the heart rate.

3. Touch

Touch can be a powerful therapy to all people all the way from babies to elderly. The belief is that even a single touch can help heal. This is evident from the various massage techniques used to calm and soothe newborns and infants. There are many nursing homes that use touch therapy an integral part of the ways nurses and staff provide care to their residents.

Have you ever felt down and depressed and depressed, yet a gentle handshake or an embrace from a loved one eases your pain away? Touch can heal. It can give you the sense that someone is caring. It is a feeling that runs through someone's heart. It communicates many emotions, including the warmth of love, affection and trust.

4. Balances your energy

The pressure applied to various points on your body can help your body experience the optimal level of homeostasis. Massages clear pathways and balances energy flow throughout your body.

5. Lets you enjoy ultimate peace

The pressure applied to reflex points within your body relaxes the organs which are associated with these points. The feeling of relaxation results from the more supple blood flow and energy circulation in your body. Your nerves will also relax and, in the end improve your overall health.

6. The effects of healing

It also has positive effects that many have experienced. It can help alleviate headaches and migraines. It alleviates discomfort and inflammation. It also helps reduce the signs that are associated with PMT and kidney disorders. It helps in lowering your blood sugar levels and aids in improving your digestion health. It also helps reduce the feelings of feeling of anxiety that people with dementia is often experiencing. It also helps the gall bladder and thyroid.

Chapter 8: Key Tips and Strategies

It's easy to learn reflexology. It is helpful to make a diagram of the reflexology to make use of as a reference when you are following the methods that people who are new to reflexology can perform easily. The following chapters will instruct you the fundamentals on how to apply reflexology on your feet or face, as well as the hand. Before you can learn the specificsof reflexology, here are some aspects you need to be aware of about this type of alternative therapy.

1. It is not advised to massage those who have been in bed for longer time than 24hrs. If they've only recovered from certain ailments and have a low tolerance to pain, they are not yet high. If they ask you to continue with the massage, make sure you are gentle. Make sure to pause frequently and ask whether they aren't injured by the pressure you're applying.

2. A good session should last for longer than 30 minutes, subject to the body's age and build that the person is. If you're

attending to an infirm patient, older person or still young, it's not recommended to extend the session beyond 30 minutes.

3. This is best to perform the entire body massage rather than just focusing on certain pressure points, according to the health issues that the person suffers from. Do the entire massage and then spend more time applying pressure where the pressure points that are related to the health issues of the patient are.

4. If you are learning to perform reflexology, it's recommended to start with the feet. It is likely that you will find written research and studies on this kind of reflexology because it is practiced widely in many countries around the world.

If you've already perfected the techniques, you are able to quickly apply the reflexology technique to different parts of your body.

5. It's not a good idea to make use of massage oils or creams for reflexology. These products can assist in relaxing and

soothing the nerves of the patient however, they can make it difficult for you to apply pressure to your fingertips. The skin is slippery. If you are planning to apply the products, it's best that you apply creams and oils after the massage. Let the scent and effects of these treatments to stay on the client to aid to relax him in the following massage.

Instead of creams and oils alternatively, you can use baby powder or talcum when you're performing the massage. Powders absorb oils in the body of the person and allow you to apply the pressure you need. Sprinkle the powder on the hands and feet of the patient before beginning the massage. It is also possible to choose the powder that has a pleasant aroma that will help your patient relax during the massage.

6. If the patient is diabetic, request for a blood sugar levels prior to starting and then when you're done with the treatment. One might experience a dramatic change or drop in blood sugar

levels while using this type of alternative treatment.

7. You must learn the correct techniques you must employ when applying pressure to different body areas. For instance the best method to apply pressure to the soles of your feet is to walk with the thumb. You can make circular movements with the index finger to massage your hands in order to help make the pressure more firm and more deeply.

8. The person conducting the reflexology as well as the person receiving should be at ease throughout the entire session. It is possible to let the patient lie or sit, based on their preference. If you're doing the massage, be sure to do it in the angles that you are comfortable with. The massage will reflect back on the way you massage If you feel uncomfortable or uncomfortable. When performing the exercises to improve your technique, it's best avoid bending your knees and avoid putting any pressure on your knees.

9. There are different reactions to an reflexology session. Some people simply love the experience and want to relax. While others might get sleepy. Patients also display physical reactions following or during the massage. This includes the cough, burping spasms, and even a flinch. There are also cases of fatigue and fatigue after having completed the first treatment. You can reduce these reactions by reminding the patient drink plenty of fluids prior to and after the massage. Keep an extra bottle of water on hand during massage sessions and remind patients to drink water whenever you want.

Chapter 9: The Foot Reflexology Chapter

The first thing you need to master in conducting foot reflexology is practice of thumb walking. You can practice this for a long time without straining your hand. The principle is easy. Your thumb will move forward by bending it and then it will come back to a point of bending.

The first step you must do is to work on your thumbs. Take a look at the top of both thumbs by placing your two opposite each other and looking them over. The tops on your fingers until your nails are nearly touching. The point where the two thumbs meet is used for the massage.

Practice using a pen when practicing the method. You can hold it in your hand. Utilize the thumb of the other hand to touch the pen using the area which was mentioned earlier. Bend your thumb, then let it straighten and repeat the procedure. While doing this, make sure the pen doesn't move and that your thumb remains in contact with the pen. This is the place where pressure comes from.

The pressure will be felt when your thumb is straight and allow the fingers to move forward while it is bent. Begin slowly. Once you've mastered the art of it, you'll be able to practice the technique in a more rapid manner. It is also possible to practice it on similar surfaces like chairs and tables. This method provides a an extensive treatment to your feet.

Begin with the Foot Reflexology

Always begin your exercise with the correct foot. Draw a diagram of the foot reflexology process to assist you to find the pressure points on your feet. These are the steps to finish this.

1. Massage the foot to relax it by massaging the foot slowly. Start from the toes and work your way up to the heel. Repeat this exercise for 30 minutes or until you feel the muscles begin in relaxation and loosen.

Cover the area around the spine of the foot using the palm of one hand, then grip the foot's bottom with your thumb of the other hand. Make a gentle twist while gently wringing your hands away from each other. Repeat this for about 30 minutes.

2. Start by focusing on the thumb walking through the foot's spine. Begin by working from the heel up to the toes and work downwards from the toes toward the heel. Work starting from the left and moving to the right from the back until you've completed the whole foot.

3. Keep the toe that is larger in your hand and gently turn it gently. Repeat this motion to the other toes until you're done with the one that is the smallest. While you are rotating attempt to stretch the base joint which connects the toe to your foot. This action affects the skull bones. It can be believed to be beneficial in relieving headaches.

4. Find the meridian points of the toes. They are found at the bottom of the toes. They are not located on the middle finger. Then, you apply pressure to the meridian point of each toe, making an arc. Toes are moved in a clockwise direction for 10

minutes before moving it counter-clockwise for 10 seconds. Begin with the largest toe and move on until you're finished with the smaller.

5. Begin your thumb-walking exercise on the toes. Start moving upwards, starting from the base up to the tip, in an unbroken line. Continue this motion until you're done with the toes on all sides. The pressure should be strong, yet soft.

Be aware that there are some people who's toes are extremely sensitive. Try experimenting with the pressure, and ask their preferred pressure. Do not lose the firmness the pressure. It can irritate the patient if you only apply pressure gently.

6. Massage the ball of your foot and refer to it in the chest area. Make the massage gentle upwards, downwards and with an angular motion until the entire area is completely covered.

7. Do the same on the back and top toes. Start from the toes up towards the ankle, then work starting from the right side to the left side of your foot.

8. Check out your diagram and see where the waistline is found. It's the thinnest region in the lower part of the foot. Its position may vary from person to person. The thumb walk covers the entire foot which is related to the stomach and liver.

9. Then, you will do the thumb walk in the region that lies between the pelvic region as well as the waistline.

10. Massage the pelvic region, which is the area that corresponds with sciatic nerve. Perform the motion starting by starting from the left, moving to the right and then up until you are towards the back of the heel.

11. Once you're done, massage your whole foot in a relaxed and gentle motion for at least one minute.

Now you are finished with your right foot. Repetition the steps, but this time, focus using the foot on your left side of the patient.

Be sure you have water to drink throughout the session. Instruct the patient to drink an ounce of water prior to you begin. This will allow the blood cleanse of toxins in the body. It is recommended that patients continue drinking plenty of water throughout the day following the treatment.

Chapter 10: Face Reflexology

Face reflexology can be administered by yourself however, you are also able to do it for others. Before you begin, be sure that you've printed out a chart of face reflexology to allow you to identify the areas that you should focus on.

Learn about the 15 points of the face. By applying pressure to these points, it can boost circulation, which is an excellent method to unwind. It is usually recommended for those who need to relax and relax from the stress they face daily.

Use your thumb or index finger to apply pressure on areas of the face that have reflexes. Simply push your finger towards the pressure point and then turn with the fingertips without lifting it. Perform the motion in the same place thirty seconds of counterclockwise motion, then 30 minutes in an reverse direction.

When performing this type of reflexology, it's best to ensure that the person who is receiving the treatment sits. The head and shoulders must be supported fully. Follow the steps behind your patient in order to allow the patient to walk.

Below are some steps for how to accomplish this:

1. The reflex points should be stimulated in the face one at a. Use a diagram to apply pressure to the points in a sequence. You should work on the entire face first, then focus on and then apply pressure to specific points.

2. Tap the area under the eyes with the tips of your fingers. two hands. Taps should be soft. Tap from the nose up to the ears. Massage the jaw line with two hands, beginning at the top of the ear, up to the chin. Place your index fingers on the chin and start rubbing the chin for around 15 minutes. Move your fingers away from the chin towards the edges of your mouth, until you are at the cheeks. Massage the cheeks in a circular fashion for about 30 minutes.

Place your fingers on the forehead, nose and then apply pressure to the eyebrows by moving your fingers with an outward direction. The fingers should be pulled upwards until they reach the hairline. Apply pressure to this area, then do the same thing on your scalp. You are free to be as active as you wish in this region as it is very soothing.

3. To reap the maximum benefits from this method of reflexology, make sure you remind your patient of the importance of drinking water. It is essential to allow your patient to drink water prior to your session and in the time following that. The patient should stop and rest after the session is finished.

Chapter 11: Understanding

Reflexology

What is reflexology?

Reflexology can aid in relieving physical pain as well as help reduce the psychological aspects of illness like anxiety and depression.

What is reflexology and what does it not?

Treat or cure any disease. Reflexology isn't the solution for cancer or for the typical cold. But, as cold remedies are utilized to treat effects of the cold it is also possible to use reflexology to ease the symptoms of certain illnesses.

Although it isn't known to treat or cure any condition, reflexology has been acknowledged in the Mayo Clinic as an effective means of alleviating pain and stress for patients suffering from many illnesses and ailments. It has been practiced as a method of alternative treating symptoms since the days in the time of ancient Egyptians. There are many reflexologists who are certified however, reflexology is an option you can practice at home.

Before you can begin to practice reflexology at home it is essential to be aware of the concept and how it can be used to treat physical and psychological pain relief.

What exactly is reflexology?

When we talk about reflexology, we refer to the process of applying pressure to certain parts of the hands, feet, or even to the ears. It is a kind of massage for therapeutic purposes that is based on the idea that there are pathways connecting the feet, hands and ears that connect to other areas of our body by which we can channel positive energy that heals us.

The use of neither oil nor lotion is employed in this practice, and the method by which you apply pressure is dependent on the location you are trying to treat. The theory is that specific areas of the feet, ears and hands, referred to as reflex spots, are connected to limbs and organs on the body. The proper way to massage the areas of the foot, ear or hand in a proper method is believed to alleviate pain in these areas of the body.

This type of massage is usually done using thumbs, fingers, and palms. However, it can also be done by pressing, stepping or rolling the feet and hands against beads or stones. Beaded foot massagers operate by utilizing this concept. For hand reflexology, small balls such as golf balls could be utilized similarly with amazing impact.

Certain areas are identified and you may have used a type of reflexology and not even know the way you're doing it. One of the most popular home remedies for relief from toothache can be to rub the region in between your thumbs and forefinger. This technique is based from the same principle as reflexology, but the points of reflex for sinuses and teeth can be located located in an entirely different part of the hand, based on contemporary reflexology charts.

The effects of reflexology can be a simple treatment to ease symptoms for many. But there are some who do not need reflexology and it is advised and could be risky. If you are in one of these categories, you should not follow the recommendations in this book , or consult a qualified reflexologist.

* Women who are experiencing unstable pregnancy

* Individuals who suffer with deep vein thrombosis, or thrombophlebitis

* Any person who has an infection that is severe and feverish

* A person who has cellulite on the hands or feet

* Anyone who recently had stroke

* People who have bruises, cuts and swelling. blisters on feet, hands or ear

Others who need to consult a physician prior to considering reflexology, and only do it by a trained professional:

* Women who are in the first trimester of pregnancy

* Anyone taking an anticoagulant medication

* People who are suffering from cancer

* Diabetics who need insulin

Anyone who has an infectious condition

* Anyone who suffers of chronic fatigue, fibromyalgia, or another illness that triggers extreme sensitivities

* Anyone suffering from epilepsy.

* People who have had heart surgery in the last few days.

Reflexology Basics

Refer to the chart

To ensure that reflexology will be effective, it is necessary to first understand the specific regions of your hands, feet , and ears that correspond to the proper parts of your body that you would like to focus on. The book's next chapter are three reference charts to serve this goal. If you are only dealing with just one area or two that need pain relief, you can focus on these areas now and concentrate on learning other areas when different ailments arise.

If you look over the charts, you'll be able to see that the zones for feet and hands are quite alike. If you place big thumbs and toes, and wrists and heels, you'll notice that the zones are in a similar way, with just some minor variations. For instance the spinal zone on the hand extends through the center of the inner edge of the thumb to the point the point where the wrist starts. On the foot, this zone is found at the inner edge of the foot. It begins at mid-section of the large toe, and running into the middle of the heel's side. This means that if you've identified the position of zones from the foot map, you'll be able easily find the zone that corresponds to it on the hand, or the reverse.

Learn to move

Also, you must know the fundamental techniques to know the proper way to massage each part of your body. In certain situations this may require only a few times of pressure. Sometimes, a turn of the finger that is massaging is all that is required. Another method, referred to by the name of thumb walking involves the use of either thumb to "step upwards and downwards across the area using the thumb to press down and then return up.

Thumb walking is a common practice for to work on the foot's most sensitive areas and also the greater areas that are the hands. Pressing with rotation is usually most effective for the toes, fingers, and the palms of your hands, and certain tiny reflex points, like beneath the foot's ball are best stimulated by constant, steady, and hard pressure for a period of 15 to 20 minutes. Similar to any massage, whatever feels best will usually be the most efficient. If you feel like you're easing the pain of a muscle, then you probably are performing it in the right way. If you attempt one approach but it isn't comfortable Try a different method and see if it is more comfortable for you.

What tools are used in trade?

In general, the only tools required are the thumbs, fingers and palms, however other tools can be employed also. Small balls, smooth stones beaded rollers, pebbled pathways may all be employed to induce results from reflexology. They can be particularly beneficial for those who want to do DIY reflexology, but don't have the flexibility to reach their feet using their hands. They can also be helpful to those who might not have enough the strength of their grips because they can use balls to exert pressure instead of using their thumb and finger strength.

Instead of lotion or oil cornstarch or talcum powder can be used to facilitate movement and stop sweat from forming.

What should you expect when reacting

Depending on how long or intense the session may be and the amount of tension that has been created in the area or the way your body's wiring is and positioned, you could get a myriad of reactions following and during the reflexology session.

These reactions may include however, they are not only limited to:
* We are laughing
* Crying
* Fatigue
* A rise in thirst
* Flatulence
* Feeling cold
Feeling lightheaded
* Sweating
* Coughing

* Sighing
* Belching
Minor muscle spasms

Chapter 12: Getting Started

If you've learned the basics, you're ready to prepare for your first reflexology session. If you're performing reflexology for yourself or a person you know, it's important to prepare the area ahead of time especially if you're just starting to experiment with the methods. You should choose the ideal location and room for your reflexology session and also ensure that the tools you need are on your disposal when you require they. Also, you must ensure that you're at ease, even if you're performing the exercises on other people.

The location for your session is supposed to be cool and peaceful. It is important to create the space in a way which encourages relaxation. Therefore, dim lighting could help. Incense or candles that smell of incense, as well as gentle, soothing music aren't necessary but they could help to make the space more tranquil and suitable for healing.

If you're working your reflexes, ensure that you are in a comfortable spot to lie down or sit. It is suggested to sit up when you are unable to reach your feet. So, you can roll your feet across the ball without the risk of falling. If you're massaging another person, ensure that they have a comfy place to lie down or sit and also that you have a comfy, easy-to-moved location to sit in while you massage their hands, ears and feet.

Take your chart as well as any talcum powder or tools you might be employing and keep them to hand. Before you begin to tackle yourself taking an honest self-assessment. Do this by making an inventory of every illness and complaint you've had issues with lately like headaches, heartburn and insomnia, pain etc. It is important to list them by importance so that you can begin with the most severe ailment, and progress to the most common symptoms. Consult your charts whenever required to ensure you're targeting the areas that are needed.

If you're doing the treatment on someone else take a break and ask them questions about what their physical ailments are. You might want to note down the answers so that you are able to focus on the various areas of pain. Similar to making your list of complaints, let them rank the complaints according to their importance.

Before you begin the session, be sure that they are not in the categories previously mentioned for those who shouldn't undergo reflexology. There are serious complications that can occur for these groups of people, especially if they are using reflexology. The most important thing you do not want is for your loved one to be admitted to the hospital due to the blood clot that was in their foot.

If you are practicing on your own or demonstrating the techniques to someone else, before you begin, spend a few minutes calming yourself before starting. Begin by being comfortable in your chair. Close your eyes, and take several deep, slow breaths in through your nose , and to exhale through the mouth. If you're supporting someone else in need, let them take the same steps.

The foot Reflexology Chart Map
This chart shows the most important reflex points of the foot. The charts may not be identical, since certain charts will have less or more zones, however these are the fundamental zones and can be a great beginning point for those who are just beginning to learn the art of reflexology.

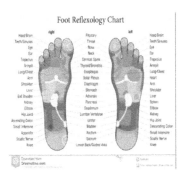

Diagram of Hand Reflexology

The Ear Reflexology Chart Map

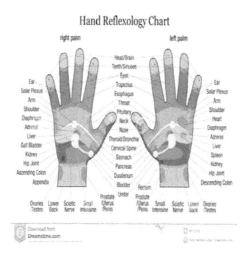

Hand Reflexology Chart

right palm   left palm

Head/Brain
Teeth/Sinuses
Eyes

Ear — Trapezius — Ear
Solar Plexus — Esophagus — Solar Plexus
Arm — Throat — Arm
Shoulder — Pituitary — Shoulder
Diaphragm — Neck — Heart
Adrenal — Nose — Diaphragm
Liver — Thyroid/Bronchia — Adrenal
Gall Bladder — Cervical Spine — Liver
Kidney — Stomach — Spleen
Hip Joint — Pancreas — Kidney
Ascending Colon — Duodenum — Hip Joint
Appendix — Bladder — Descending Colon
Ureter — Rectum

| Ovaries /Testes | Lower Back | Sciatic Nerve | Small Intestine | Prostate /Uterus /Penis | Prostate /Uterus /Penis | Small Intestine | Sciatic Nerve | Lower Back | Ovaries /Testes |

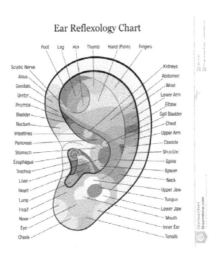

Ear Reflexology Chart

Self-Practice using Foot Reflexology

Follow the steps under How to Get Started before you begin your practice such as choosing a suitable location creating and grading an inventory of your ailments and preparing your tools and charts. Spend a few minutes to calm yourself with deep breaths prior to starting.

If at any point in the exercise, you start to feel tense or overwhelmed, allow yourself to relax and relax. Close your eyes, and then breathe slowly through your nose and out through your mouth for a couple of times, until tension is released the muscles.

If you're able to draw your feet into the lap of your sofa, adhere to the guidelines for using your thumbs and fingers to massage your reflexes. If you're not able to bring your foot into your lap or you do not have the strength of your fingers to exert sufficient pressure, then follow the methods of the balls massage method.

If you are doing foot reflexology on yourself the best to do it sitting down. The practice of foot reflexology can be performed in a chair, couch, or even on either side of the bed (as long as your feet touch the ground, if you're employing the ball technique).

Finger and thumb massage

Focusing on the areas you identified during your self-assessment start with the most troublesome part. Utilizing your chart, if you need to, locate the correct location of your foot. By using the thumb-walking method to rock your thumb towards the area of concern and press firmly but not so far that it causes discomfort. Move across the entire zone at least two times, taking two minutes or more in the most severe or large regions, or around 30 seconds in smaller zones and minor issues. In areas where pressure is required instead of thumb-walking, apply pressure to the area for 20 minutes. Release, repeating the process twice. Should the problem is bilateral, or the region has been found on both feet this on the opposite foot.

Massage ball

Place the ball 1-1.5" across, in the front of your chair. Place your feet above the ball and then lower it until the proper space is in the ball. Take a firm step by your feet and then roll, rock or press the ball on your area till the whole area has been massaged duration of 2 minutes for most difficult areas as well as 30 second for the smaller ones. When you apply pressure only press and hold at least 20 seconds. After that, then release and repeat the process twice. Repeat the process on the opposite foot as required.

Chapter 13: Practice Self using Hand Reflexology

It is a technique that can be done anytime and without having to make a plan in advance. If you're working or in the car , the theatre or some other location you are able to apply this gentle massage. It can help ease discomforts that could be triggered when you're not able to enjoy an entire session. It can be done in a sitting position or lying down. Bathing is a great location to practice this kind of self-reflexology.

Of course, to perform this procedure in public, you'll need to either remember the map, or keep a smaller version on your person. It is probably best to remember only the regions that you are likely to need when traveling, like the reflex points for the neck and head for those who are susceptible to suffering from headaches.

Similar to the self-practice of foot reflexology for hand, it may be practiced using fingertips and thumbs of the opposite hand or by using small balls.

Whatever method you choose, the guidelines are similar.

Find the region on the chart that corresponds to the area where pain is. Utilizing your fingers, thumbs or ball, apply pressure to the area that corresponds to the correct area of your body. It should take between 10 and 20 minutes, depending what size the area. Repeat the process on the other side when is necessary. In areas such as the thumb's base that direct pressure isn't appropriate, use a thumb walk or roll the ball across the area between one end and the next.

Self-Practice using the ear Reflexology

It is possibly the most simple method for DIY reflexology. Like hand reflexology, it can be performed in any location, with the privacy and comfort of a home even should you not want to do a comprehensive approach and use your entire ear, this will require you to master the zones and keeping a notepad on your own.

It is possible to do this either lying down or sitting up. It is possible to do it in the bath but particular care must be taken to avoid getting water in your ears.

With the thumb and fingers on one side, rub the ear area that corresponds to the area of concern shown on the chart. Apply a firm, rolling motion. Make sure to apply the pressure but do not press down. Massage the area between your fingers and your thumb or by placing your fingers over the attached regions of your ear for 10 times. Repeat until you've felt relief or have been massaged for one minute, or until you have reached the end of your massage. Repeat on the opposite side, if the discomfort is bilateral.

Five Do-it-yourself (Do it yourself) Reflexology Techniques for the ailment

Here are a few easy methods to treat a number of common illnesses, using self-directed reflexology. If you're unsure of the location of the zone or reflex location is you can look at the diagrams to get a better understanding.

1. Helping lower back pain and sciatica

As we get older lower back pain may become a regular issue for most of us, and especially when we've suffered an injury to our lower back previously. When Sciatic nerves are injured and the pain can extend to one of the hips.

The treatment for back pain can be expensive and time-consuming. If the pain isn't severe, we'll just have to endure it and do nothing to ease the pain apart from taking over the prescription pain relief.

Reflexology is a different method to treat the muscle spasms and pain in the lower back and the sciatic nerve.

Method of Foot

The zones that connect to lower back as well as the sciatic nerve are situated on the lower portion of the heel as well as the line that defines in the center of heel respectively. If you're self-training using the ball method, you can use it to roll across this area beginning by moving from outside your foot towards the inside, every two to three times per hour across both feet. You can also ask someone else to thumb walk over the upper back area of the heel from outside to inside, two or three times per foot across both feet. Repeat this process on the line to the nerve of sciatica. If the pain has not relieved, repeat the procedure another time.

Hand Method

The zones that connect to lower back pain and the sciatic nerves are located on the wrist, and not in the palm itself. The sciatic nerve is the contour of the bottom of the palm, where hand meet wrist, and the lower back zone comprises the whole region that extends for an inch or just below it - but with the exception of a small circular space to either side, located below the palm.

Ear Method

There isn't a reflex point zone in the ear that connects to lower back, however the spinal region is located just beyond the opening of the canal of the ear. The sciatic nerve is located in a tiny space that lies close to the front curve in the front of the ear. Use a straight pin that has the head of a ball and then press an eraser on the sharp end of the pin to ensure safety and then push the ball into the areas by making a bouncing motion for the spine region and then turning with a firm force for a few seconds in the area of the sciatic nerve. Repeat the procedure for the other side of the ear, in case the pain is bilateral.

2. Stress and tension are relieved.

Tension can build up within our bodies when we're stressed out or stressed about things. This can result in tight muscles that can cause headaches and other issues. The reason why this happens is due to the fact that our brain sends signals to our nerves creating defense mechanisms that can cause our shoulders as well as the other parts of our bodies to slump and tighten, to prepare for the fight or flight response. In order to reduce tension, we must focus on the nerve centers of our bodies. They are situated in the brain and spine. The use of the reflex points in these regions can also assist in relieving discomfort of headaches.

Method of Foot

A reflex zone of the spine begins in the outer part of the toe that is the largest on each foot, and extends downward towards the outer border of middle heel. The toe's edge corresponds to the cervical spine, and so on and the outside heel's edge representing the sacrum. The brain zone and head extends across all of the of the toes, where the pad is located, with the exception of the big toe where it extends to about half way across the pad of the big toe.

Utilizing your thumbs or a ball apply a rotating force on both the sides of every of your toes, one at a moment on both feet. Begin with the largest toe, and then work towards the outside. You can then either thumb walk or roll it across the inside of your foot, starting at the in the middle of the big toe, and moving downwards until the middle of the heel. Repeat this on the other foot. Do this three times as often as necessary to lessen tension.

Hand Method

The reflex point area on the hand, which is linked to the spine, runs from the middle of the outer part of the thumb to where the wrist's beginning point is. The head zone is located on the pads of the four fingers, and on the upper part of the pad that is used that is for thumb.

By rotating the pressure of your thumb or finger apply pressure to each finger tip in a separate way, beginning by rubbing the thumb. Work toward the pinky finger. Repeat the same process on the other hand. Then, the thumb should be walked across the outer edge of the thumb to just below the palm on the wrist. Repeat this on the opposite hand. Repeat this three times until the tension eases.

Ear Method

The ear's spinal zone is just outside of the opening to the canal of the ear. The brain zone is located near the top of the earlobe located on the side that is closest to the head. Move your head along the spinal region of each ear by using an ear ball with a straight head, with the sharp edge, capped with an eraser to ensure safety. Carefully but gently massage the reflex point of your brain with your thumb and your forefinger.

3. Combating fatigue and increasing energy and alertness

There are many reasons you might feel tired and not at the level you want to be. Maybe you didn't have a restful night prior to going to work, perhaps your children have left you exhausted and it's several hours before they are put to bed. Or maybe you're planning a long journey. Whatever the reason, fatigue can be anything from annoying to hazardous.

The use of reflexology could help combat fatigue by targeting different glands that control energy and parts of the body that are related to breathing. This means that we be able to get more oxygen and help us stay alert. The adrenal glands as well as the thyroid glands are responsible for combating fatigue and keeping alert and focused. The solar plexus as well as the diaphragm are responsible for regulating our breathing , and help us feel more relaxed and focused on our work.

Foot Method

The reflex points that correspond to the glands of adrenal are situated near the center of your foot. It is situated on a diagonal across the first two toes to out to the side of the feet, where the base of the largest toe joins. The zones for the reflex point for the solar and diaphragm can be found underneath the sole of your foot. The solar plexus zone lies nearly directly in the middle of the line and directly towards the toe's second. the diaphragm area is the line running underneath the ball.

Utilizing your thumb, finger or ball method Apply pressure direct to the middle point of your toe for around 20 minutes, then let it go and repeat the process two times. Apply this pressure to both feet. Then, using your fingers thumb, or a ball and move along the lines of the thyroid area by walking or a rotating motion, beginning on the outside of your foot, and moving inward. Repeat this several times. Repeat with the opposite foot.

Then, insert your finger into the region that is the solar plexus, and push upwards for 20 minutes. Release and repeat the procedure twice. The thumb should be walked across the bottom of the foot's ball beginning from the outer side and moving to the inner. Repeat the process twice. Repeat the process in the other direction.

Hand Method

The reflex points that correspond to those glands of the adrenal are situated close to the middle in the palm. Thyrotoxic reflex points lies just below the bottom knuckle the thumb, which is located just above the fleshy area on the palm. Solar plexus reflex is situated just below the pad of middle fingers. The diaphragm follows the outline of the pad of the three fingers.

Utilizing your finger press the palm by alternating the palm in the palm's center. For 20 seconds, apply pressure to the palm and then let it go. Repeat the process two times. Repeat the entire process in the opposite direction. Utilizing the thumb of the opposite hand, move it through the bottom of the knuckle of your thumb, starting from outside, and then work inside. Repeat this two times. Repeat this process in the opposite direction.

Place a finger in the palm, turning to the left, just below the your middle finger.

Continue to rotate the finger for 20 minutes. Repeat the process twice, and then stroll across the line for the diaphragm. Repeat the process with the other hand.

Ear Method

There are no areas in the ears to these regions.

4. Improving depression

For tackling depression through reflexology, we must focus on the reflex points for the pituitary gland as well as the hypothalamus that regulate mood, as well as those areas of the body that are linked to breathing in order to increase the amount of oxygen in our bodies, an endorphin releaser that is natural. Stimulation of the solar plexus as well as the diaphragm reflex areas can aid in making us feel more focused and on our health.

Method of Foot

The area that is associated with the hypothalamus and pituitary gland is situated dead within the middle on the big toe of each. The reflex point zones of the diaphragm and solar plexus are located beneath that ball in the toe. The solar plexus area is nearly directly in the middle of the line while the diaphragm forms the line that runs beneath the ball.

Place your thumb in the reflex point of the pituitary gland, and apply rotational tension to rub the region. This should take about 20 minutes. Release the pressureand repeat it twice more. Repeat on the other foot.

Then, place your finger in the area for the solar plexus . Then push upwards for 20 minutes. Release, repeating the process twice. Take a step with your thumb across the outline of the foot's ball starting from outside and ending on the inside. Repeat this two times. Repeat both steps with the opposite foot.

Hand Method

Place your thumb in the reflex area for the pituitary gland that is located on the thumb. Apply the thumb with a steady, rotating press to rub the region. This should take about 20 minutes. Release the pressureand repeat the process twice more. Repeat the process on the other side.

Put a finger on the palm and rotate it little, under the middle finger's pad. Continue to rotate the finger for 20 minutes. Repeat two times, then move across the line to the diaphragm. Repeat the process in the opposite direction.

Method for Hearing

There aren't any corresponding zones in the ears to these areas of the body.

5. Insomnia and fighting it

There are many causes for insomnia. If you're not sure about the root of your difficulty to fall asleep then the best approach to address the issue is by massaging all zonesinstead of trying to concentrate on just one. This is to relax all the zones and provide you with more chances of sleeping.

If you know the root of your insomnia like stomach or stress It is possible to target the areas in the feet, hands and ear and address the issue immediately. If not, follow the guidelines listed below to focus on all body parts and induce relaxation.

The foot massage works best when you have an assistant If not you can try the method of ear or hand or do the foot massage while you are in the bath. Warm bath water "tricks" the brain to believe that your thumbs and fingers aren't yours and will make the massage more efficient.
Method for Foot
Beginning with the largest toe begin by massaging the pads of each toe gently in circles. Continue to massage until you've massaged your entire toe. From the big toe, move towards the outside of the foot, until you've massaged your pinkie toe. Then, you can walk your thumb along the outside of the pinkie toe , and across the outside of your toe, including its cushioned portion.

Begin to move along the outside of your foot until you get to the heel. Massage the heel from the outside edge of the foot to the inner edge to the inside of the heel. Follow this by walking with your thumb through the inner side of your foot until you reach the top of your big toe.

Move your foot across the sole of your foot Pay attention to every area until you've reached the area you've previously massaged. Continue to work up and across until you've stimulated every reflex point within the arch of your foot.

Take a break and allow yourself to do your breathing exercises. Repeat the same process on the opposite foot.

Hand Method

Starting with your thumb, gently massage the length of your fingers with the opposite thumb and finger until you reach pinky. From there, you can massage the outside of your finger between your thumbs and the forefinger. By rotating your thumb into small circular motions, move over your wrist, across it and then back to the pad near the base of your thumb, and then across the lower portion of the padded area. After that, work your way through the unpadded portion of the palm. Focus on the areas that are not massaged until all reflex point zones are massaged.

Do a few seconds of repeating the breathing exercises, and then repeat the exercise on the other side.

Method of Ear

You can work on only one ear at time or both ears simultaneously depending on what is the most efficient and easiest for you.

Starting with the earlobe Start by rolling the ear lobe's skin the ear between your forefinger and thumb starting from the lower part of the ear until the top. Once you've worked the ear's lobe and the an ear's shell, beginning at the head and then working towards the head, move around the inner reflex points that surround the ears in an opposite direction until all the zones are covered.

The Hand Reflexology Method: Specific Tips and Methods

Hand reflexology is great for public areas, if it isn't possible to complete a full practice of reflex points on the feet.

* Try using zones of relaxation in your hands when you are on phone calls with angry customers, or in similarly tense

situations when you fear that you could become angry and make a mistake.

* Try to copy the reflex points onto your hands for the first time you attempt the technique, to assist you in trying to identify which zones are. Alternately, you can make multiple versions of the charts, minus the labels, and then write zones on the blank charts. This will assist you in working towards being capable of filling them in all on your own without having to reference the chart.

The hands should be soaked in warm water prior to your massage session can not only help to relax, it will also aid in your ability to massage your reflex points for longer , without feeling tired.

* The talcum powder and corn starch assist in massages and stop sweat from causing friction on your skin, however, it can get messy. Keep an clean dry towel in your fingertips whenever you're performing an exercise session, whether alone or with a partner.

*The amount of time you spend on sessions with reflexology is entirely up to the frequency you prefer. It is possible to schedule lengthy sessions every week, or schedule smaller sessions daily. You can try small sessions during the most stressful hours during the day.

* If you must keep at the very least one hand free however, you still have a need for the relief reflexology may provide, place an object on the desk or table and gently roll your hand across it, putting pressure on the zones that need it.

* Unless the area only is present on one hand, you must apply the reflex point to both hands. However, this exception is where the pain is exclusively on one part of your body. Also when you feel your left shoulder is hurting just massage the area that is for your left shoulder, not the right shoulder.

Foot Reflexology: Specific Tips & Techniques

* Whether you're self-practicing or doing the art of reflexology with a partner be sure that the feet clean and dry prior to you start.

* Socks are a good option to wear in a reflexology session in place of the talcum powder.

Although you are not able to concentrate on particular regions of your foot or specific reflex points however, it is possible to stimulate every point walking along a walkway with pebbles.

* Reflexology exercises in the bathtub is possible even if you aren't able to reach your feet and require balls. Simply hang the ball by using string in order to play with it using your feet.

* If you're unable to reach your foot , and you do not have a ball that you utilize to massage your reflex areas, then you may also make use of the rounded edge of an object like chairs for the outside points of your foot, as well as any object with an edge that is rounded to help to reach your feet without bending. For example, the edge of a broom handle.

Another method to stimulate all the reflex points in the feet at the same time is by filling a dishpan with marbles, then move your feet over them.

* In the case of muscle pains it may be helpful to massage the reflex points which connect to the nearby parts within the body. For instance If you're suffering from shoulder pain it could be beneficial to work on the zones on your feet that are connected to your neck and arm.

Ear Reflexology: Specific Tips & Techniques

* To locate the most tiny reflex point areas within the ear place an eraser on the sharp edge on a straight pin using the ball head. Use the ball to move the region.

* If the space isn't too tiny it is possible to employ the eraser tip of the pencil and massage your reflex points.

* Cleanse the outer layer of the ear using the help of a cotton swab, dipped into rubbing alcohol prior to starting the ear reflexology treatment.

* Do not place the ear with talcum powder or apply it to your fingers while manipulating areas of the reflex points of the ear.

* As the areas in the ear area are tiny and unique in comparison to the feet and hands, and can't be discerned, it could be

best to have a friend to help. However it could be that you consider it beneficial to take an overall approach and massage your entire ear to ensure that all areas are treated.

Chapter 14: What's Reflexology?

Reflexology is a process that involves applying pressure to specific zones on your hands, feet, or ears. It is generally relaxing and could be a good way to reduce tension. The idea behind reflexology is that these zones are connected to the body's system and organs. People who practice reflexology believe that applying pressure to these areas can benefit the overall health of the individual.

Reflexologists use hand and foot charts to guide them when applying pressure to particular areas. Sometimes, they utilize things like wood sticks, rubber band or rubber balls, to assist their job. The majority of reflexology practitioners are physical therapists, massage chiropractors, and physiotherapists in addition to other.

Research conducted by researchers from the National Institutes of Health and the National Cancer Institute indicate that reflexology could improve relaxation and sleep, and could help reduce psychological symptoms like anxiety and depression.

Research has also shown that reflexology can aid in the care of cancer patients.

Reflexologists also assert that the practice may assist in the treatment of various ailments such as diabetes, cancer and asthma. However, studies that support these claims are not sufficient. There are more studies in the pipeline. Although generally accepted as safe but when performed in a vigorous manner - could cause individuals to feel uncomfortable.

While reflexology hasn't been recognized as a medical practice in the world but thousands of alternative practitioners have used it for a long time and have achieved good results. In the event that there exist alternative treatments to treat more than 12 medical issues that affect various areas in the human body, wouldn't an acupuncture session or two worth a try?

Reflexology Using Reflexology

The effects of reflexology are different for each person who makes use of it. The theory is that it is a relaxing response of the body. Hands that have been trained to be sensitive might detect changes when touching their hands, feet or ear. They also can detect small deposits of soft tissues of the body.

Reflexology gently nudges the body to allow it to work better by enhancing the flow of lymphatics and venous circulation. It also promotes relaxation, stimulates nerve pathways and assists the body correct itself.

A further discussion of the benefits of reflexology will discussed in the future.

Because reflexology is a treatment for your body's needs in an holistic way, not just a disease's specific symptoms, a lot of individuals can profit from the practice. As we've mentioned it's suitable for the majority of people even people suffering from specific medical conditions.

This is because the duration and pressure are adapted to satisfy the patient's specific demands. Reflexology could be beneficial for:

* Reducing tension and stress
* Helping to relieve pain

* Acute and chronic illnesses
* Improved the supply of blood to nerves and improving nerve function.
* Revitalizing energy
* Homeostasis (balancing the whole system)
* A preventative treatment
* Children and adults of all age groups
* Inspiring the body's ability to eliminate the toxins and impurities

The considerations are necessary for infants, children and the sick and even the older. In these instances the session with a reflexologist should be shorter and the pressure should be less. Certain clients are advised to consult their doctor to determine if reflexology is appropriate for their particular situation.

The benefits of specific conditions are:
* Sinusitis
* Sciatica
* Hormonal imbalances like PMS
* Sleep disorders
* Digestive disorders
* Mild depressive disorders
* Anxiety

A full reflexology treatment involves treating all pressure points on both feet. The session may last between thirty to sixty minutes according to the style of practice and the level of wellness of the client. In a reflexology treatment the patient might be experiencing:

* Tingling or Twitching
* A desire to rest and a sense of deep relaxation
* Warmth to the body part being addressed
* Feelings of the body expanding and expanding when it relaxes.

A brief discomfort that could be due to the body's regions of imbalance

Medical professionals and practitioners who specialize in complementary medicine generally agree that a large number of the body's health problems can be attributed to stress. A body trying to function under pressure will not be able to repair injuries and protect itself from disease.

Stress can be physical emotionally, mentally, or even environmental.

Reflexology is principally a relaxation therapy that can help reduce the effects of stress and aiding the body to be in balance and to let go. By using reflexology your body is able to better manage the stress caused by illness and the demands of daily life.

A Short Introduction to the History of Reflexology

It's difficult to determine the origins of reflexology given how old it is. It is believed that reflexology was first introduced to been transmitted through oral transmission. It is believed that the practice of reflexology, as well as other medical procedures could have been first documented in a picture in 2330 B.C. at the Egyptian tomb of Ankhamor.

The reflexology symbols are widely believed to be written on Buddha statues feet throughout India and later in China. In the Yellow Emperor's Classic of Internal Medicine (1,000 B.C.) includes a chapter about the examination of feet and also the first of discussions in print about the relationship between the feet's zones and points as well being the vital force.

In the year 1300, Marco Polo was believed to translate into Italian an Chinese massage book. Hence it was believed that he introduced massage and reflexology into Europe. In addition, a book about reflexology's fundamental element, called zone therapy written by Drs. Adamus and Adamus was first published in Europe.

The United States in 1917, William H. Fitzgerald, M.D. is regarded as the father of reflexology wrote about 10 vertical zones running across the body's length. He found the application of pressure to an area that was related to an area of injury could be used as a means of relieving pain for minor surgery.

The Dr. Shelby Riley expanded on Dr. Fitzgerald's research. The Dr. Riley developed a map of horizontal zones that run throughout the entire body. He also created maps of reflex points in the feet and hands. The doctor. Riley also suggested pressure points in the ear's outside part.

A close associate to the Dr. Riley, physiotherapist Eunice Ingham, was also prominent in the development of reflexology's modern. Through her research on pressure points In her research, Ms. Ingham observed that her feet were most sensitive and responsive. She created foot maps (still being used to this day) and in 1930, she introduced the principles of reflexology to people outside of the medical field. In the International Reflexology Institute, Ms. Bingham conceptualized one of the most widely used chart of reflexology, which has since been revised to accommodate Dwight Byers, her nephew.

The Dr. Paul Nogler, in 1954 recorded a map of reflexes of the points in the outer ear. Dr. Nogler's work was further developed through Oleson as well as Flocco. Research maps are currently being taught as an integrated method of hand, foot and ear reflexology.

Reflexology's Benefits Reflexology

The benefits of reflexology include improving energy levels, stimulating the function of nerves, increasing circulation cleansing contaminants by stimulating the central nerve system, removing urinary tract issues that cause migraines, alleviating anxiety and sleep disorders, improving recovery time after surgery or injury, and bringing you into a relaxing state. It can also aid in dealing with certain cancers more effective. It can also ease pregnancy pains and even pains that occur following the birth of the baby.

A lot of people are on their feet for the entire working. If your job is in the field or factory, office, in a hospital or at any other place of work it is likely that you're putting pressure and weight to your foot on a regular basis. Stress may also manifest elsewhere in the body.

It is the same about back discomfort. In the case of back, people visit a masseuse and receive massages, so it's only natural that there should be a massage for the feet too. Reflexology could be described as an exercise for the feet, but there's more than it is. It is a distinct form treatment, reflexology covers the hands and ears which makes it more than an ordinary foot massage.

While reflexology is primarily utilized to ease stress, it may also aid other parts of the body to function properly.

Energy Levels. By coordinating the functions of various organ and muscle systems reflexology can boost energy production and metabolic processes in the body. If you're feeling tired and in need of some energy, a session can help you get more energy to accomplish what you have to complete.

Nerve Function. As you age the nerve endings get less responsive in specific areas such as the extremities. Reflexology is believed to be responsible for stimulating more than 7,000 nerve ends during one session, thereby stimulating nerves functioning and reactivity.

Cleansing and opening of neural pathways can increase the flexibility and function of numerous areas of your body. These neural paths are comparable to muscles, so it's a good idea to exercise them (via reflexology) periodically to ensure they're in good condition.

Relaxation. Reflexology is a method to open neural pathways. The result of this free-flowing action is a relaxed body, with a decrease in stress levels. It will help you relax by bringing calm to your mind and across your body. It may also aid in overcoming sleep problems like insomnia that can be a problem for those who need to rest enough.

It assists your body to settle into a more relaxed state and return to its normal cycle of normal circadian rhythms.

Circulation. One of the benefits of reflexology is to improve the overall circulation of the body. This means that blood and oxygen flow through the body at a higher speed. The more oxygen is able to reach the organs that are vital; thus improving organs' performance. This means that metabolism is enhanced. A healthy circulation - with the aid of reflexology can also lead to faster growth and the healing to damaged cells.

The stimulation of nerves. The open neural pathways can benefit to improve the functioning of your nervous system a variety of ways. Through reflexology, brains can efficiently handle inputs, meaning that cognitive functions will improve. Also, memory will increase and physical reactions will become quicker and fluid. The brain will generally be more efficient and quicker.

Elimination of Toxins. Reflexology can help ease urinary tract problems and enhance the functioning in the bladder. Reflexology helps eliminate contaminants as well as other foreign substances and also help shield the body from a variety of ailments and health issues caused by the urinary tract that is not functioning correctly.

Improves healing. The combination of improved nerve and circulation, and the metabolism's equilibrium results in cells being able to regenerate more quickly and wounds will heal faster. Reflexology's benefits for relieving pain will make people feel more comfortable in a short time. They also are willing to begin physical rehabilitation so that they can get back in the world.

Migraines and Headaches. A lot of people utilize reflexology to alleviate discomfort. Reflexology, as an anti-inflammatory treatment, can help reduce migraines and headaches' intensity. It does this by easing muscle tension which is often the cause of these conditions. The headaches that are caused by stress can be eliminated because stress and psychological factors are often reflected in physical symptoms of migraine.

Before you decide to take the Tylenol, perhaps you could try the reflexology treatment for your headache. Also, you'll be at peace afterward.

Menstruation and pregnancy. Studies have shown that reflexology can help pregnant women, especially with regard to the duration of labor and need for analgesics in the post-partum recovery. It may help decrease the chance for a new mother developing post-partum depression. It also helps the body recover faster, so that it can quickly return to normal metabolic activities.

Relieves the symptoms of Cancer. Although reflexology isn't an alternative to treating cancer, it may help alleviate cancer treatment's (chemotherapy) negative side negative effects. It aids patients in reducing anxiety and help them sleep better. It also eases the vomiting and nausea that is caused by cancer's treatment procedures.

The effects of reflexology that are more general such as increasing circulation as well as clearing the neural pathway can help slow the spread of cancer cells as well as increase the action of antioxidants that can be beneficial in the destruction of cancerous cells. But, research is in progress regarding this.

Although much of the research into reflexology hasn't been widely accepted, the stories of successes and thousands of people who have used traditional methods are not to be discounted. Many people continue to use reflexology as a treatment option. This is why reflexology should be considered more of an alternative therapy for medical ailments.

Reflexology is completely safe, and isn't harmful using it in conjunction with conventional treatments of ailments. Make sure to find an experienced reflexologist to help you with. With time, you could be able to apply certain self-reflexology methods that you will find useful.

Chapter 15: Reflexology Chart Maps

Before beginning to practice reflexology It's best to learn about what alternative therapies are connected to it. There are many of them like acupressure and Acupuncture. It is comparable to these treatments in that it alters the vital energy of the human body by stimulating certain points in the body. Acupressure/acupuncture points, however, do not coincide often with the points that reflexology uses.

Acupressure and reflexology are considered reflex therapies because they utilize pressure points in a specific area of the body that influence different parts of the body. Reflexology uses reflexes in a way that resembles human body shape around the hands, ears and the feet. However, Acupressure makes use of hundreds of reflex points on meridians (thin energy lines) which run throughout the length of the body.

Massage is another form of therapy that is similar to reflexology. Both therapies are often interchangeable. Both massage and reflexology make use of touch, their techniques differ.

* Reflexology employs the use of the reflex maps of regions and body points within the hands, ears and feet by employing micro-movement techniques such as thumb-walking or finger-walking as well as hooks, with the goal of creating an energy response all over the body.

Massage is the fundamental manipulation of your body's soft tissues using specific techniques such as friction, the stroking, kneading, or tapping to loosen muscles.

Massage therapists operate from the outside in order to manipulate certain muscle groups in order to relieve tension. However the reflexology practitioners work from the inside out for stimulation of the nervous system to ease tension.

In order to practice reflexology efficiently The therapist should have an understanding of all maps of reflexology that show foot (the most popular map) hands, hands, and ears. Therapists can access these points on the feet and hands (top, sides and the bottom) and also the ears (both inside and out to the extent that they can be accessible) to influence organs and systems across the body.

Maps of reflexology have been circulated across the globe by practitioners. There is no consensus about the points between reflexologists. A general consensus, however, exists regarding the main reflex points. Also, there is scientific evidence of the linkages between inner organs as well as the surface of our skin.

To illustrate how the body's systems relate to one another Reflexologists use'reflexology charts. The most popular reflexology map is that of the feet. Each foot is representative of the vertical part that is the body.

The right foot is a reference to the right side of the body and the organs that reside on this side. The liver, for instance is located situated on the right side of the body so its identified reflex spot is situated on the right foot.

• The foot of the left is connected to the left side of the body along with all the organs and valves are located there.

A reflexologist can conduct an all-encompassing session, or focus on a specific area of concern in the hands, ears or feet. If there's no time, and the client is looking to relax for instance, the practitioner can focus on the ear. Whatever techniques they employ the reflexologists believe that they're working on releasing the nerve system's congestion or stress by stabilizing the energy flow of the body.

Beginning to Learn About Reflexology

If you're considering trying at relaxing with reflexology or even to complement any therapy you happen to be taking, you must be aware of what goes on during the regular reflexology treatment. In addition, you need to be aware of what its main principles are.

The body responds to contact which may aid in multi-level healing. Clients of reflexology may often believe they must 'concentrate or focus to enjoy the benefits of this practice. Although calmness can bring about more profound feelings, you do not require any special techniques or abilities to be successful. If the practitioner is aware of what they is doing, permits energy flow to take place, and remains in the present, the client may react.

It is the body's natural healing process. reflexologists are only assisting in this healing process. Instead of acting as the healer the reflexologist is merely an active participant in the session. It is crucial for practitioners to center and ground themselves , and then let the client heal themselves.

It is a recognition that reflexology's purpose is to assist in the balancing of the person so that the body can restore and nurture its own body. The practitioner is aware that reflexology's goal is to assist the patient align their self-healing and energy flow.

Practitioners and clients may feel energy moving. A reflexology practitioner might feel the energy flow of pressure points on the hands or feet, as well as the ears and feet to the rest the body. When treating the gallbladder and the spleen, for instance the reflexologist is able to feel energy flow and also access the points at the exact at the same time. Due to the power of these two points clients can also feel the flow of energy.

Human beings comprise an physical and emotional body along with a mind and spirit which are interdependent. The reflexologist examines every aspect of the client's existence the mind, spirit emotions, body, and mind. Relaxed bodies can lead to peace of mind, a harmonious spirit and calm emotions.

Once you have a better understanding of the underlying principles that underlie reflexology, you can learn the process of the reflexology session. The typical session starts with the practitioner conducting an assessment of health to determine whether that is actually the best method of treatment.

The practitioner will explain to you how reflexology works and the process that takes place during the reflexology treatment. He also informs you it is not a medical substitute and it is not able to treat any specific health issue. There are also some doctors who may require for you to fill out a consent form form or consent form. Once you've signed the form the session begins.

Based on your specific medical condition depending on your particular health issue, the reflexologist could choose to focus on just the hands or ear, or feet. There are also certain instances when a patient in a hospital may receive an acupuncture session for food, even if they are connected to multiple IV tubes as well as other tubes and wires.

It is best that the reflexologist decides what type of treatment is being performed on you. If the therapist decides to treat your feet, then you'll lay down or sit and fully dressed, with the exception of your shoes and socks. The reflexologist will clean to soak and massage your feet then put them on her/his chest to the level of your chest.

The practitioner will begin by checking your feet for any sores, open wounds, rashes, plantar warts, or bunions and will also inquire about any foot or leg discomfort that could hinder treatment. As we mentioned previously the duration of a reflexology treatment ranges between 30 minutes and an hour. If you wish, you can rest or talk during the therapy session. You'll still reap the benefits of the treatment even if you sleep during the session.

While the session continues it is recommended to give feedback and you are able to have the reflexology session stopped at any point in case you experience discomfort.

The Reflexology Treatment

A full therapy session employs different techniques, and incorporates reflex points of both feet (maybe even the hands and ears). The session of reflexology begins with the fingers or toes, and then moves to that heel area of your hand or foot and then moves to on the sides and top of the area that is being treated.

The reflexologist, through applying pressure to the pressure points, addresses the internal organs and glands, as well as the muscles, bones and nerve ganglions (brachial and solar the plexus) as well as sciatic nerves throughout the session. If congestion or tightness are discovered during a session the reflexologist applies pressure to bring the body into balance.

If there is an area that causes discomfort, the area is worked on until the location or point achieves harmony. The relief from pain should not be the aim. Instead, it helps bring the human body back to equilibrium which means that pain will disappear. The nervous system is stimulated to complete the work. After the session is over the therapist will return to the location or spot to determine that the pain is gone or it is not.

The Session is over

A lot of reflexologists offer a type of tranquil and serene way to end a session. This involves stroking the hand or foot and keeping the limb in a certain way. It is crucial to feel pampered and soothed. It is equally important to be relaxed throughout the session.

Do not feel pressured or rush to complete things after the session has completed. Relax and return slowly towards the moment. Once you're relaxed then slowly draw yourself up to go out feeling refreshed. It is recommended to drink plenty of fluids and stay conscious of your body for the coming hours. In case you've got any questions or concerns it is always possible to call for your physician.

While in a session, you might experience some reactions. A lot of these reactions are a sign that the treatment is working. A few of the signs that typically last for up to a couple of days indicate the body's effort to return to the state of harmony and equilibrium. The symptoms could include:
* Improved sleep
* Energy levels increase
* Additional mobile joint
* Pain relief
* Tiredness
Kidney stones are easily transported

* Spots, pimples, or skin eruptions (due to elimination of toxin)
* More the amount of mucus (vaginal ou nasal discharge)
* Diarrhea, frequent bowel movements (toxin elimination, cleansing)
* Release of emotional or psychological tension (crying)
* Flu-like symptoms

Mandatory Sessions

The number of sessions required is different and is typically determined by the reason of the person to seek reflexology as well as the health of the person. The results of reflexology sessions are subtle and cumulative therefore, it would be best to schedule more sessions, ideally every week for 2 months.

If you're suffering from a particular condition such as illness or a condition, then you could require additional sessions. The most common recommendation is to begin with a single each week session for up to six weeks. Following that, you continue with a each month's session.

It is not a diagnosis

A lot of people believe that a reflexology treatment is diagnosis of a particular health issue. No, it's not. Reflexologists don't tell you about any congestion or tension they might find on the ear, hand or the foot during a session of reflexology that might indicate any anomalies.

One of the theories behind reflexology is that the body can heal and nourish itself after stress is relieved. When your body's stressed, it could be referred to a different therapy or a medical team at any time it is necessary. The reflexologist is not able to diagnose a condition or give out medical recommendations.

Reflexology Techniques
With its long and storied history long history, it's no surprise that reflexology is an alternative treatment that has numerous strategies and techniques. Both the West as well as the East have created their own unique styles of reflexology which are efficient. Innovative techniques and methods are rapidly evolving as reflexologists across the globe create and

share their findings and experiences from clinical practice.

The Ingham Method

Created through Eunice Ingham, who was a physiotherapist. The Ingham Method is the basis for how contemporary reflexology is performed. Ingham is a physiotherapist who developed the method. Ingham is regarded as the "Mother of Reflexology' by many reflexologists. In the Ingham method the pressure is applied using the 'thumb-walking.' In this way the thumb or finger is bent and straight while maintaining an unchanging pressure on the hand, foot or ear region which is being treated.

The practitioner makes use of talc. A particular session could last for one hour, based on the health of the client. The primary goal in Ingham Method Ingham Method is balancing the system of the body as well as to help promote relaxation. The practitioner works with the patient's tolerance to pain. In the holistic reflexology treatment the reflexes of all types are worked on , with some being treated more than other.

Rwo Shur Method Rwo Shur Method

In many regions of Asia particularly the areas of Singapore, China, and Taiwan The Rwo Shur reflexology method is in use. It's a mix of thumb-sliding techniques and pressure and incorporates the knuckles . It even small wooden sticks. The therapist applies hard pressure and applies cream to create an efficient, fluid, and quick movement.

The sessions typically last for one hour, and is focused on stimulation, not relaxation. In Taiwan this technique was created by Fr. Joseph Eugster, a missionary from Switzerland. After having experienced firsthand the benefits of reflexology the Fr. Eugster realized the need to assist those who needed help with the simple reflexology technique. He began to treat and instruct others on this particular type of reflexology.

Ayurvedic Reflexology

This form of reflexology that is based upon the principles of Ayurveda, is defined best as a successful blend between Western and Eastern practices and theories. Ayurveda is India's complete traditional, ancient, and traditional medical system. Reflexology that is based on Ayurveda gives practitioners a thrilling innovative approach to the foot and hand. Sharon Stathis, in Australia invented the method that is regularly practiced in at least 15 countries.

The Ayurvedic Reflexology method is designed to maintain the balance of the body's subtle energy systems by encouraging the prana's (vital energetic) efficiency. Prana moves through the body through Nadis (micro energetic channels). According to Ayurveda doctrines both the body and the mind are not well if prana's flow is disrupted or slow.

The nadis is lined with the marma spots (energy centers) which help maintain prana flowing at its best. Marma points are located on the vital nadis within every hand and foot. The whole body benefits by working on these points.

Ayurvedic Reflexology foot and hand sessions.

It is vital that the therapist use oil when working on points of marma, as any friction that is not needed could upset the delicate balance of energy. In Ayurvedic Reflexology Sesame oil, which is warm, is often utilized. The best type of oil is one that is not bleached and organic. It's also non-deodorized and cold-pressed. It provides the practitioner with an lubricant to work on Marma points. It is also an best base for brisk and flowing moves associated with this type of therapy.

Ayurvedic Reflexology could be more gentle to the hands of the therapist than the standard thumb-walking method of reflexology. The process, in general, is fast, but it results in a complete relaxation. In this session, every hand or foot is completely treated. A therapy of Ayurvedic Reflexology may last 40-45 minutes.

New Methods

In recent times in the West the reflexology community has been looking for ways to control and balance the body's subtle energies using the feet and hands. Acupressure techniques and points that are linked to energy treatments are employed more often during a reflexology session.

The ancient Chinese wisdom is the foundation for new ideas where study of the principles of the yin/yang principle and The Five Phases Theory, and meridians are applying holistic treatments to new heights. Magnets, special oils, and colors in a torch form can be applied to reflex points. The majority of practitioners incorporate gentle touch that connects reflexes in order to promote balance and an energy flow.

Although they are not novel, ear and hand reflexology are increasingly used alongside foot reflexology. Practitioners can use the ear, hand, or foot reflexology together in one session. They can also select the area of reflex they believe is appropriate for the client. Reflexologists are currently being trained in different techniques and techniques. That means that reflexology practitioners can offer you the right session for the specific needs of your.

Chapter 16: Reflexology to Weight Loss

With increasing rates of obesity and, as a result serious health problems like the type 2 diabetes and heart diseases becoming increasingly common and commonplace, people are becoming aware of the importance of taking control in their overall health. There's a growing pressure to stay slim in the midst of a world that seems impossible, especially when you're confronted with processed, processed fast food that's loaded with fat, but lacking in nutrients.

The battle to lose weight is a huge challenge for those constantly fighting it. However, there isn't any quick solution to losing weight over the long run So, you should put the weight loss pills aside and put away your pre-packaged diet plan meals. You have to alter your way of life, gradually by making better choices in all aspects of your lifestyle, from food to exercise to even how you think. The positive thing is the fact that you can find efficient and natural supplementary methods and programs that could assist you in losing the extra pounds. And reflexology is just one of them.

Making healthy choices

The loss of weight does not only affect your appearance from your exterior, it also affects also how you appear and feel inside. The prevalence of obesity is increasing all over the globe And all this extra weight that we carry around could lead to serious health problems, such as cancer, heart disease, and diabetes. If you're overweight when you're pregnant and have a child, you both risk being confronted with both long-term and short-term health problems.

Don't panic! There are many options to get your weight in check. The most important thing is to not think about doing any of the fad diets or fasts that the majority of celebrities are trying. If you're looking to shed weight, it's crucial to make adjustments to your lifestyle which will last the long haul. A lot of people who shed weight following an extreme exercise or diet plan, find themselves putting the weight quickly when their routines change (and everyone has to modify our routines at one time at some point or other).

The secret to losing weight effectively is to make healthy choices. Begin to pay attention to your diet and replace the unhealthy foods you've been eating with healthier alternatives. A visit to a nutritionist can be an effective method to help you get started to achieve this. In addition, you should add a little exercising into your routine. It's not necessary to become a bodybuilder however, you can go down the stairs time instead of using the elevator. Also, make an effort to take 30 minutes of exercise every day.

Give Reflexology a Try

If you've decided to make healthier lifestyle choices Try reflexology! A nutritious diet and a dose of regular exercise paired by reflexology is an extremely effective method to help you lose weight. Reflexology methods to lose weight can be performed at home, by yourself or if you wish to ensure you're getting the most efficient results, consult an experienced reflexologist. A professional reflexologist may assist you in preparing the right diet plan to go to your reflexology sessions to lose weight.

What is the process?

The reflex areas on your feet and hands which correspond to digestion organs, the spleen thyroid system and the nervous system. These points must be identified to regulate your digestion, metabolism and energy levels. This can help your body burn greater calories and calories. If you stimulate your spleen, you'll also be less hungry and satiety, which is a beneficial technique to shed weight.

Simple Methods to Lose Weight

If you're considering trying the reflexology method to lose weight by yourself there are several important areas of your body that you should focus on. The stomach, spleen and gallbladder, pancreas and the endocrine glands are all components that comprise your digestion. These when stimulated will perform more efficiently and to lose weight.

For starting out to begin, you'll require charting of the reflexology foot and hand such as these:

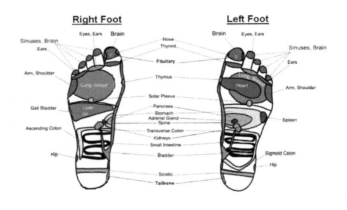

Hand Reflexology Map (palmar side)

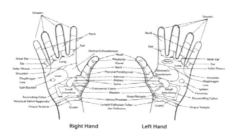

Right Hand   Left Hand

Each exercise should be accompanied by the reflex point of the hand or foot that is in line to the area of your body that you'll work on. The exercises should be performed at a rate of 5-10 minutes daily every week, five times and should be completed alongside an appropriate lifestyle and fitness regimen.

Increase the Spleen's activity to reduce the Hunger

Invigorate the spleen reflex by placing your left foot and placing it in your right hand, and then employing your thumb on the left side to stimulate the area of the reflex. The same process can be done with the palm.

Stimulate Stomach as well as the Pancreas to help absorb more nutrients.

Invigorate the pancreas and stomach by placing your left foot with your right hand, and then press the reflex points in that area with the left hand. Move your thumb towards the outer edge of the reflex zone and then switch feet. Repeat the exercise using your palm.

The Gallbladder to emulsify fat

Utilize the same method as for the pancreas and stomach to activate the gallbladder reflex on the palm and foot.

Increase your Endocrine Glands to Regulate Hormones, Appetite, as well as Stress

Make use of your thumb and concentrate on applying pressure on the thyroid reflex point and adrenal glands and pituitary on your palm and the foot.

Chapter 17: Reflexology to Eliminate Tension and Stress

Stress: We've all felt it in the past. Even the most calm and balanced people can be overwhelmed at times it's perfectly normal because it's a natural phenomenon. It's your body's reaction to good and bad experiences , but when you're dealing with prolonged stress, your overall health can take a huge drop and your health could be at risk in a variety of ways.

The effects of long-term stress on your Body and Mind

If you live a hectic life with a lot of obligations at home, as well as an extremely demanding job to top everything else, it could be extremely detrimental to your body and your mind. Stress that lasts for a long time can also be caused by a variety of events and circumstances such as physical ailments or traumatizing circumstances, divorce, death or other similar situations.

Chronic stressors like those can have a negative effect on overall health as well as wellbeing, and if you do not adopt measures to keep your stress in check it is possible to be faced with a variety of health problems that could affect your quality of life and cut valuable years off your life which include:

* Anxiety, depression and irritation
* Headaches
* Insomnia
* Eating Disorders
* Substance Abuse

Increased chance for developing Hypertension and other problems with blood vessels

* Higher risk of suffering from stroke or heart attack
* Acid Reflux
* Stomach issues like nausea and/or constipation, vomiting or diarrhea.
* Bodyaches, especially back and shoulder discomfort.
* For women with irregular menstrual cycles can be seen.

* In males with lower testosterone levels can cause impotence or Erectile dysfunction
* For men testing, the urethra, testes and prostate are more susceptible to infections
* More prone to contracting colds, flu and other viruses
* Higher risk of contracting infections and illness
* Speedier recovery from injury or illness

You can clearly see that negative psychological and physical consequences of chronic stress can be severe. However, how can manage the effects of stress when there's many other things to think about?

Effective Strategies for Reducing Tension and Stress

If you live a hectic lifestyle, it's vital that you take action to bring the stress out of your system before it causes things more detrimental to your health. It is crucial to learn to appreciate your own health and quality of life enough to elevate your physical and mental well-being up the list of priorities for the day. We often neglect the health of our bodies until something more serious occurs, but you should not do this. When you had a trusted acquaintance Wouldn't you have helpful advice to pass on? Do it yourself and take an eye on your health.

There are a variety of various techniques you can use to lessen stress. It is possible to begin by creating your daily routine and sprucing up your diet as well as exercising more and experimenting with meditation techniques in the evening and in the early morning as and breath exercises during the entire day particularly when you're in the center of a stressful situation. These techniques can give you an increased sense of calm and control and inner peace.

Utilize Reflexology Techniques to Get Effective Stress Relief

There are certain reflex points in your forearms, hands, and feet that help reduce tension when you press and press them. The practice of massaging these points for a few minutes is particularly effective when it's in conjunction with breathing exercises to ease tension and stress. You can massage these points by yourself whenever you're stressed or before bed at night.

Utilize the forearm to control the heartbeat, ease your mind and body, and increase circulation

The forearm point is situated on your wrist, in between the tendons running through the inner part portion of your forearm. To locate that sweet spot determine the length of your thumb multiplied by two, extending to in the forearm's middle, from the line between your wrist and hand. The reflex point is located here between the tendons and then knead it using small circular motions. There will be a slight sensation of pain that is comfortable when you're performing it correctly.

This reflex point aids in relieving and treating insomnia, heart palpitations, nausea and vomiting.

Make use of the wrist points to relax your mind and ease your body.

It is possible to find a reflex spot on the opposite the wrist's left or right at the junction between your wrist and forearm. It can be effective in calming the mind and relaxing your body when it is used correctly. Place the point on the wrist's end close to the bone of your wrist. Knead this reflex point with the same motions that you made on your forearm.

This reflex point aids in reducing insomnia, heart palpitations, emotional turmoil and memory problems.

Make use of the foot to ease tension, relax and sleep better

If you take a look at the foot chart from chapter one, you'll observe the point at the foot's bottom in the lower regions that are connected to the breast and lungs. Place that point on the inside of the foot until you feel a slightbut comfortable sensation of pain. Keep the point in place for a couple of minutes and repeat the process on the opposite foot.

In addition, you can look up the foot and hand charts found in the first chapter of this book. They work on the reflex points of the kidneys, spleen and heart and the liver. These organs are intimately linked with stress and anxiety and it is suggested to treat these areas if you are looking to relieve energy from these zones.

Chapter 18: Reflexology to Treat

Pain Relief

When you're exhausted, sick or suffer injuries, the muscles tighten up and can cause a great deal of pain and tension throughout your body. What do you think of those random back and neck aches as well as intense pains that do not end, regardless of how many times you massage and rub the region? If rubbing and kneading the sore spots aren't doing the trick, and taking medication doesn't work, there are numerous methods and treatments to help reduce discomfort.

Ease Your Pain Using Effective Reflexology Techniques

Techniques for reflexology are highly effective in relieving pain in the back shoulders, head, and neck, resulted from stress, exhaustion or minor physical injuries. The technique relies on applying pressure and pressing, or massaging areas of the feet and hands that correspond to the neck, spine and shoulder shoulders.

If done correctly When done properly, these techniques can be extremely efficient in relieving mild discomforts and aches. However, it is important to note however, that they are unlikely to be effective for relieving the severe discomfort caused by injuries that are serious or, in the long run severe pain. If this is the case, talk with your physician about combining the reflexology treatment along with your regular treatment. It will at least help alleviate stress and will surely take tension and pain away!

Reflexology for mild Back Pain

If you've been on feet for hours, made it through a strenuous exercise, or simply exhausted the reflexology methods can significantly ease back pain.

Utilize the foot chart from chapter one to find the reflex point of the area of the spine in the inner part the foot. Use your fingertips of the hands to secure your foot with your thumbs at the bottom and your fingers on top. Slowly and gently move the hands opposite ways. Do this for only 30 seconds to unwind.

After you've completed the relaxation method, use the thumb of your hand to "walk" across to the point of spine reflex. Begin at the bottom of the heel , and then walk your thumb upwards until you reach the top of your big toe. Repeat from the tow up until the heels. Perform the same technique however, instead of moving on the ground, you should press with a vertical motion going down the inside of your feet.

Do the thumb walk two times, and end your exercise using the relaxation method you started with. Repeat the exercise with the opposite foot.

Reflexology for Shoulder Pain and Mild Neck Pain

If your shoulders start to hurt after a long working day or you experience a sharp pain when you work do this technique to relieve the discomfort.

Begin with the horizontal thumb walk that we discussed to help with mild back pain. Start with the right foot.

Once you've finished this thumb-walk, follow the chart found in chapter one to find your reflex points on your foot that connects with the neck. Perform the thumb walk along the reflex point. Move between up and down and diagonally. Repeat this process a couple of times.

Locate the reflex point which corresponds to the shoulders. Then, perform the thumb walk the same manner as you did to the neck area. Repeat this on the top of your foot, in the same point that corresponds to the shoulders. After that you can gently massage the bone's notch under your tiny toe at the outside of your foot. Repeat this for approximately 30 minutes.

Once you've completed the exercises listed on your right foot, do the same exercises on your left foot.

Reflexology to treat Headaches

Headaches can be uncomfortable and painful and they can be frustrating and distracting. If you are suffering from headaches and require quick relief, try a basic reflexology treatment.

Then, put the palm of your finger on stomach to provide support. Next you can use your index finger and thumb to gently grasp the joint at the base of your thumb. This is the point which is where your thumb joins your hand. Massage the joint by rolling it in one direction to create the full circle, then continue to move to the other direction.

Then, you can shift your fingers upwards and keep the reflex point above the second joint of your thumb. Then, turn with a gentle side-to-side movement for five seconds. After that, make a circular motion to move around in one direction, for 5 seconds and change directions after five minutes. This is the same for every joint of each finger of the hand.

Then, place all your fingers and your thumb to massage your hand. Then, squeeze the thumb by moving it upwards and downwards and then around the entire side. Repeat this process for each finger of your hand.

Change hands, and then repeat these steps with the other hand.

Chapter 19: Treating Illness Using

Nature's cures

There have been many exciting developments in the field of medicine in the past few decades however, that does not mean that everything is well in the realm of modern medical science. Despite the advances there are many who have grown skeptical of modern medical professionals and doctors and are now beginning to search for alternative and holistic treatments for various ailments and illnesses.

Take a look at Nature to find a cure

The issue with many modern treatments that contain prescription drugs for patients is that they don't tackle the root of the health problems to solve them completely rather the majority of times the medication eases certain symptoms of the illness, while new problems result from the adverse effects of the drug. Therefore, the patient has to find a new prescription to fight those adverse consequences, and that's where the cycle starts. Certain people with cancer, diabetes, or other illnesses are taking numerous medications. However, they might find solutions in the natural world if they follow a holistic path towards healing, instead of adhering to the current medical practices.

It's not the norm for modern doctor to inquire of the patient about their lifestyle and diet when they present with a health issue However, they are the first places that one must examine. Poor diet and lifestyle can be the point at which any illness develops and, in turn, is the best place to be effectively treated.

Reflexology as a Supplementary Treatment Method

In order to successfully tackle any specific disease or illness using natural remedies, you must mix various techniques and treatments to develop an overall balanced lifestyle and diet. There isn't a single holistic treatment that can treat every ailment by itself However, when you combine diet, exercise and other treatment options to treat your particular ailment and body kind, you've got the recipe for a successful treatment that's likely to be more efficient than any other modern medicine available.

There are various herbs and food items that help heal specific areas of the body and eliminate illness as well as certain herbs and foods which should be avoided based on the condition you're experiencing. Certain exercises and holistic therapies help relieve symptoms, unblock energy and encourage cleansing within the body, which is highly effective in managing a range of ailments and illnesses.

What can Reflexology do to help?

Reflexology is a practice that has been utilized over the years to aid in healing in the body through eliminating blocked energy, promoting cleansing, and restoring balance within the body. It's best used as an adjunct treatment to ease pain and aid the body heal itself.

Reflexology can be particularly efficient in relieving symptoms that result from the following illnesses, ailments and illnesses:

* Breathing and respiratory problems

Sinus issues

* Bowel and other digestive problems result from stress
* Unbalances and irregularities in hormones
* Trouble sleeping
* Recovery after surgery
* Musculoskeletal discomfort, particularly in the neck, back and shoulders
* Nausea that is triggered through chemotherapy and other severe medical treatments
* Fibromyalgia

While reflexology isn't accepted as a standard part of modern medicine however, scientists and doctors are working hard to prove the validity of the ancient practice and incorporate it into modern medicine as a viable type of therapy. To date studies conducted in clinical settings have discovered several major health benefits associated with reflexology, such as:

* Balance and maintaining blood pressure and the immune system.

* Positive function of the respiratory system
* Pain relief for muscular and skeletal injuries and post-operative recovery
* Balance in blood sugar levels
* Improvements in the Bowel function
* Reducing anxiety levels and stress
* PMS relief as well as lower time to labor for women.
• Relief of sinus issues headaches, migraines, and sinus problems
If you're suffering from diabetes, asthma as well as anxieties, allergies or neck, back or PMS, shoulder pain digestion issues migraines, headaches, or other digestive issues Reflexology as a supplement to treatment option will definitely assist in balancing your body as well as your mind and provide the much-needed relief.

Reflexology Techniques for Illness

For the most effective treatment and treatment of post-operative discomfort and other issues that result from severe injuries or diseases visit a qualified reflexologist at minimum 4 times a week. The experts will apply the old-fashioned techniques they are proficient in and are in a position to tailor a treatment plan specifically for you, which will include nutritional and diet tips which can greatly assist in the recovery process.

However, there are some easy techniques you can apply to your own at any time to ease tension in your sinuses, swollen glands nausea and vomiting as well as sore throat. These are among the most frequent ailments due to allergies common cold and flu. Reflexology can be particularly efficient in easing these symptoms.

Help to ease a sore throat by using Reflex points on the hands

There are numerous joints and bones in the fingers and toes , which connect with the neck's top and the bones of the jaw and skull which is where you should be focusing on in case you're experiencing a sore throat.

Begin by placing your palm of one hands on the stomach to provide support. Next utilize your index finger and thumb to hold the joint at the base of your thumb. This is which is where your thumb joins your hand. Massage the joint by rolling it in one direction until you have an entire circle, and then repeat the process with the opposing direction.

Then, move your fingers upwards, and then hold the reflex point above the second joint of your thumb. Then, turn with a gentle side-to-side movement for five seconds. Then, make a circular motion to move around in one direction, for 5 seconds and change directions after five minutes. Repeat this process for every finger joint on your hand.

Finally, put all fingers and the thumb to massage your hand. Squeeze the thumb while moving it upwards and downwards and then around the entire side. Repeat this process for every finger of your hand.

Change hands, and then repeat these steps with the other hand.

Cool the Wrists for Relief from Vomiting and nausea

The wrists are crucial reflex points since they link all the energy meridians that are located in the hands to the other parts of your body. When these points are cool they cool the entire body and instantly relieves nausea.

Make use of cold water, or something else cold, such as ice, frozen veggies or a cold piece metal or a cold wall, or anything similar. You can run the water across the insides of your wrists in the area where the lines cross between your hand and arm, with the palms facing upwards. In the event that you do not have any water then place an object of cold or coldness on your wrists or place them against something cold. Repeat this from 30 to two minutes or whatever it takes for nausea to go away.

Use the toes to relieve Glands that are swollen. Glands

If you are experiencing mild swelling of the glands, you should focus on activating the gland point reflexes in the feet. The method to ease headaches, which is discussed in chapter 3 can also be efficient when applied in addition to the techniques used to treat glands.

Start by rotating the large toe of your right foot by securing it by the base and gently moving it around in circular movements. The goal is stretching and turn this joint at the base. Moving up the toe, do the same to the top joint. Repeat this motion gently for each toe.

After rotating the toe with the lowest size, do a thumb walk across your toes beginning with the largest toe. Do this by placing your thumb horizontally across the top of the toes. Make use of the chart in chapter one to identify the reflex points for the pituitary and thyroid glands. Then, take a slow thumb walk over these areas by moving your thumb in an upward direction across, diagonally and downwards. Repeat this process for about one minute.

Get rid of blocked sinuses by pressing the tips of your Fingers and toes

The fingertips of your fingers and toes are linked to your sinuses. They could be blocked for various reasons. It is a highly uncomfortable condition that makes it difficult to concentrate or think. If you are in need of quick relief from sinus obstruction Try this easy method of reflexology to improve the flow of blood through your sinuses. It will also aid in breathing again.

Use the chart in chapter one to identify the reflex points of the sinus region, located near the ends of your fingers as well as your toes. Begin by using the right thumb. squeeze the sides of your point in a continuous pulsating motion for five seconds. After that, repeat the movement at the middle of the point, near the highest tip of your thumb. Then, move towards the middle finger, and do the same thing. Repeat for each finger, and then switch hands.

The same method is to be applied to the sinus reflex points that are located on the toes.

Conclusion

After you've completed this book, you should be comfortable enough to perform some yourself reflexology sessions. It should be understanding of how reflexology is implemented and how it impacts the systems of the body for a better perspective on life and better health for your body.

Reflexology isn't designed to substitute for traditional medical treatments for your health issues However, it is an aid to more effectively manage the issues your condition can throw your way. It's also useful for helping you deal with issues that occur that aren't permanent however, they can be painful. Reflexology can be used at your own discretion and discover the method that does the best for you.

To ensure that you're getting the best results , make sure you make sure that you are in a peaceful dark, dimly lit space that allows you to focus on what you are doing. If you notice that you have difficulty in relaxing, try gentle music or candles with scent within the space. Stay at ease with your body , and take note of when your feet or hands feel less supple. This could be a sign that your body is not in alignment.

The principle behind doing self-reflexology is identical for every pressure point in your hands as well as each pressure point within the feet. If you discover that the do-it-yourself methods in this book are working for you take a risk and test other reflexes from the charts included. You'll be amazed by what the difference that reflexology can make.

Thank you for reading this book.

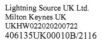

9 781774 854259